Collins

T0337072

Yorkshire Dales
Park Rangers
Favourite Walks

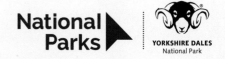

Published by Collins
An imprint of HarperCollins*Publishers*
Westerhill Road, Bishopbriggs, Glasgow G64 2QT
collins.reference@harpercollins.co.uk
www.harpercollins.co.uk

HarperCollins*Publishers*
Macken House, 39/40 Mayor Street Upper, Dublin 1, D01 C9W8, Ireland

Printed in India

ISBN   978-0-00-846265-9   10 9 8 7 6 5 4

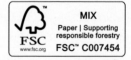

Contents

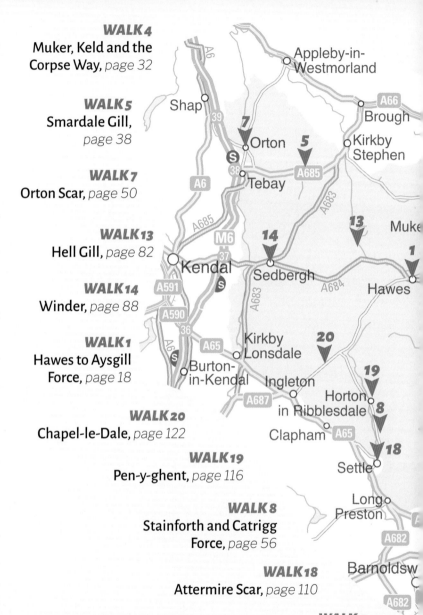

Appleby-in-
Westmorland

Shap

Brough

Orton

Kirkby
Stephen

Tebay

Kendal

Sedbergh

Hawes

Muke

Kirkby
Lonsdale

Burton-
in-Kendal

Ingleton

Horton
in Ribblesdale

Clapham

Settle

Long
Preston

Barnoldsw

WALK LOCATIONS

▼ Recommended starting point for each route – refer to individual walk instructions for more details.

Barnard Castle
Bowes
A66
Gilling West
56
53 S
Scotch Corner
A1(M)
52
Richmond
A6108
11
3, 10
Leyburn 15 A684
Bainbridge
Aysgarth
Middleham
16
Kettlewell
Pateley Bridge
9
Grassington 17
Wharfe
Skipton A59
Ilkley
A629
Embsay **Silsden** A65
Keighley

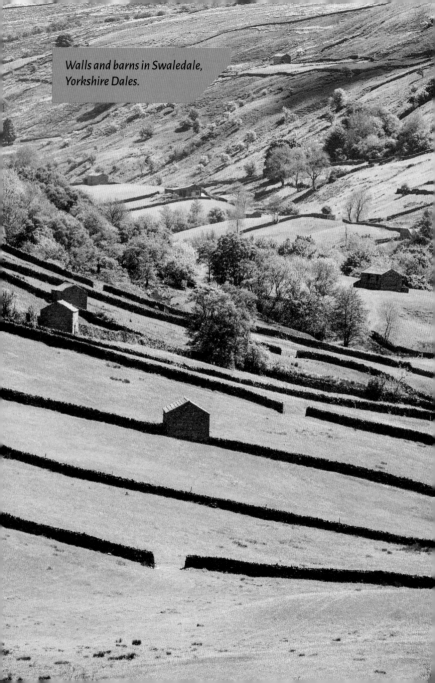

Walls and barns in Swaledale, Yorkshire Dales.

Introduction

The Yorkshire Dales has many moods; it can be wild and windswept or quietly tranquil with valleys full of hay meadows, dry stone walls and barns.

Spectacular waterfalls and ancient woodlands contrast with the scattered remains of rural industries. Together, nature and people created a special landscape of immense beauty and character – one of the most picturesque places in the country.

Whether you're coming for the day or staying longer, there's always lots going on, and there are hundreds of cosy B&B's and holiday cottages to suit everyone. Bring friends, bring family, and enjoy everything the Yorkshire Dales has to offer.

One of the best ways in which you can enjoy the Dales is by walking; so grab your boots and come and walk the Dales! There are walks to suit all ages and experience, including 'miles without stiles' accessible walks, hill and meadow walks.

If you fancy more of a challenge, there are longer distance options which include the Pennine Way, Coast to Coast, Pennine Bridleway, and the famous Three Peaks, where the aim is to walk the 24 miles, covering all three summits, in 12 hours!

Yorkshire is the home of cycling thanks to the 2014 Tour de France 'Grand Depart' and Le Tour de Yorkshire. The Dales offers some of the best cycling the country – from gentle routes in the valleys to challenging climbs over the moorland that separates them; including the iconic Buttertubs pass and Grinton Moor. Cycling here is a great way to take in the landscape and observe the wildlife. There's a network of 900 km of bridleways, by-ways and green lanes available for you to use, or you can try some of the Tour de France and Tour de Yorkshire routes. There are also plenty of picture postcard towns and villages to stop off at for refreshment.

The Dales is perfect for foodies. There are cheese festivals, farmer markets, micro-breweries, and the world-famous Wensleydale Creamery in Hawes. In every town and village there are great pubs, cafés and take away food options. Just make sure you come hungry!

The area's unique landscape character is created by the particular combination of many elements: the managed moorland, pastures and valley grasslands; small woodlands; dispersed villages and farmsteads; the local building materials; strong field patterns; and drystone walls and field barns. This is what makes it such a special place.

For example, ancient dry-stone walls and field barns are defining features of the Dales landscape, and the iconic pattern of barns and walls in Upper Swaledale is recognised as being one of the most distinctive agricultural landscapes in Western Europe. Over a quarter of England's flower-rich upland hay meadows and pastures are here – outstanding examples can be found in Swaledale and Langstrothdale – and keep an eye out for nationally important populations of birds like curlew, lapwing, and black grouse.

Livestock farming is an important part of life in the Dales. There are distinct sheep breeds like Wensleydale and Swaledale and a strong tradition of upland cattle rearing that is still deeply interwoven into local life – and made famous through local cheese making! Livestock sales and agricultural shows play an important part in the lives of local people.

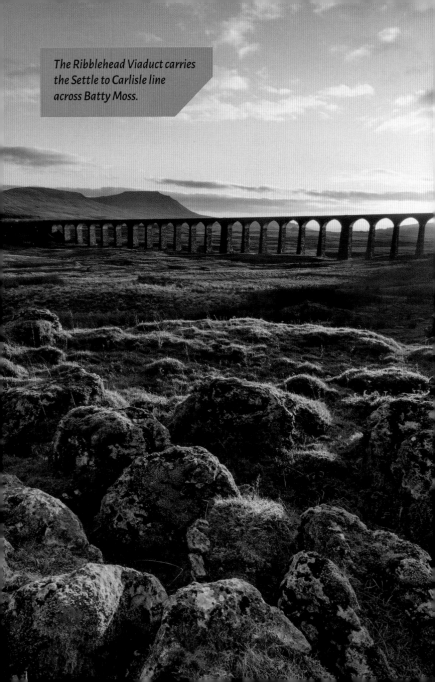

The Ribblehead Viaduct carries the Settle to Carlisle line across Batty Moss.

Some of the best examples of classic limestone scenery can be found here. With its scars such as those at Gordale and Attermire and limestone pavements such as those at Great Asby Scar and Malham Cove, which featured in *Harry Potter and the Deathly Hallows*.

There are dozens of spectacular waterfalls to explore such as Hardraw Force – the longest unbroken drop in England – Ingleton Falls, Janet's Foss and the world famous Aysgarth Falls which featured alongside Hardraw Force in the hit movie *Robin Hood Prince of Thieves*.

The Yorkshire Three Peaks of Whernside, Ingleborough and Pen-y-Ghent lie within the National Park. They're amongst the highest in the county, providing an inspiring challenge to walkers from around the world.

The most extensive caving area in the UK is here, including the longest cave system – the Three Counties System – and one of the largest caverns and the highest unbroken underground waterfall at Gaping Gill.

The stunning dark sky of the Yorkshire Dales National Park is one of its very special qualities, and each year we support a special festival to celebrate it. The Dark Sky Festival is all about discovering, learning and enjoying the galaxies and stars you don't normally get to see.

Finally, take a heritage train journey on the iconic Settle to Carlisle line which cuts through the heart of the Dales, providing stunning views of the landscape and taking in famous features such as the Ribblehead viaduct and the Westmorland fells, or take the Wensleydale Railway from Leaming to Redmire.

Protecting the countryside

Yorkshire Dales National Park Authority wants everyone to enjoy their visit and to help keep the area a special place. You can do this by following the Countryside Code.

You can find a detailed copy of the Countryside Code online at **www.gov.uk/government/publications/the-countryside-code**, but the main points can be summed up as follows:

- Be safe, plan ahead and follow any signs.

- Leave gates and property as you find them.

- Protect plants and animals and take your litter home.

- Keep dogs under close control, especially near farm animals and during the nesting season.

- Consider other people.

It's pretty easy to act responsibly when out walking. Simply take care not to disturb wild animals and sensitive habitats. Don't take things away like stones or wild flowers, and don't leave anything behind that you shouldn't. Walkers should take extra care to stick to paths during the bird nesting season between 1 March and 15 September.

Call the Yorkshire Dales National Park Headquarters on 0300 456 0030 or visit our website at **www.yorkshiredales.org.uk** for more information.

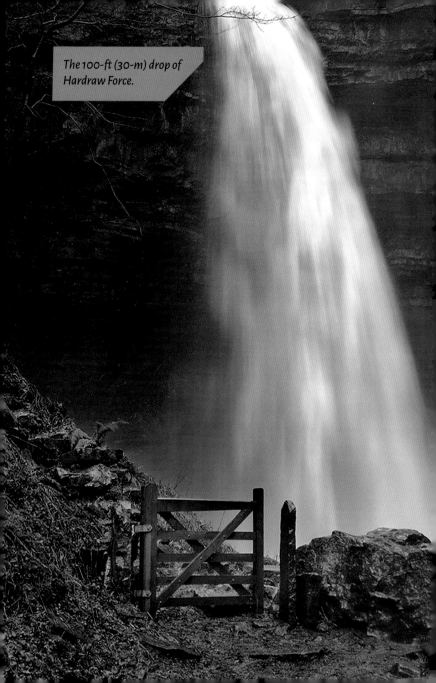

The 100-ft (30-m) drop of Hardraw Force.

Walking tips & guidance

Safety

As with all outdoor activities, walking is safe provided a few simple commonsense rules are followed:

- Make sure you are fit enough to complete the walk.

- Always try to let others know where you intend to go.

- Wear sensible clothes and suitable footwear.

- Take a map or guide.

- Always allow plenty of time for the walk and be aware of when it will get dark.

- Walk at a steady pace. A zigzag route is usually a more comfortable way of negotiating a slope. Avoid running directly downhill as it's easier to lose control and may also cause erosion to the hillside.

- When walking on country roads, walk on the right-hand side facing the oncoming traffic, unless approaching a blind bend when you should cross over to the left so as to be seen from both directions.

- Try not to dislodge stones on high edges or slopes.

- If the weather changes unexpectedly and visibility becomes poor, don't panic, but try to remember the last certain feature you passed and work out your route from that point on the map. Be sure of your route before continuing.

Unfortunately, accidents can happen even on easy walks. If you're with someone who has an accident or can't continue, you should:

- Make sure the injured person is sheltered from further injury, although you should never move anyone with a head, neck or back injury.

- If you have a phone with a signal, call for help.

- If you can't get a signal and have to leave the injured person to go for help, try to leave a note saying what has happened and what first aid you have tried. Make sure you know the exact location so you can give accurate directions to the emergency services. When you reach a telephone call 999 and ask for the police or mountain rescue.

Equipment

The equipment you will need depends on several factors, such as the type of activity planned, the time of year, and the weather likely to be encountered.

Clothing should be adequate for the day. In summer, remember sun screen, especially for your head and neck. Wear light woollen socks and lightweight boots or strong shoes. Even on hot days take an extra layer and waterproofs in your rucksack, just in case.

Winter wear is a much more serious affair. Remember that once the body starts to lose heat, it becomes much less efficient. Jeans are particularly unsuitable for winter walking.

When considering waterproof clothing, it pays to buy the best you can afford. Make sure that the jacket is loose-fitting, windproof and has a generous hood. Waterproof overtrousers will not only offer protection against the rain, but they are also windproof. Clothing described as 'showerproof' will not keep you dry in heavy rain, and those made from rubberized or plastic materials can be heavy to carry and will trap moisture on the inside. Your rucksack should have wide, padded carrying straps for comfort.

It is important to wear boots that fit well or shoes with a good moulded sole – blisters can ruin any walk! Woollen socks are much more comfortable than any other fibre. Your clothes should be comfortable and not likely to catch on twigs and bushes.

It is important to carry a compass and a map or guide. A small first aid kit is also useful for treating cuts and other small injuries.

Finally, take a bottle of water and enough food to keep you going.

Public rights of way

Right of way means that anyone may walk freely on a defined footpath or ride a horse or bicycle along a public bridleway. In 1949, the National Parks and Access to the Countryside Act tidied up the law covering rights of way. Following public consultation, maps were drawn up by the Countryside Authorities of England and Wales to show all rights of way. Copies of these maps are available for public inspection and are invaluable when trying to resolve doubts over little-used footpaths. Once on the map, the right of way is irrefutable.

Any obstructions to a right of way should be reported to the local Highways Authority.

In England and Wales rights of way fall into three main categories:

- Public footpaths – for walkers only.

- Bridleways – for passage on foot, horseback or bicycle.

- Byways – for all the above and for motorized vehicles.

Free access to footpaths and bridleways does mean that certain guidelines should be followed as a courtesy to those who live and work in the area. For example, you should only sit down to picnic where it does not interfere with other walkers or the landowner. All gates must be kept closed to prevent stock from straying and dogs must be kept under close control – usually this is interpreted as meaning that they should be kept on a lead. Motorised vehicles must not be driven along a public footpath or bridleway without the landowner's consent.

A farmer may put a docile mature beef bull with a herd of cows or heifers, in a field crossed by a public footpath. Beef bulls such as Herefords (usually brown/red in colour) are unlikely to be upset by passers-by but dairy bulls, like the black-and-white Friesian, can be dangerous by nature. It is, therefore, illegal for a farmer to let a dairy bull roam loose in a field open to public access.

The Countryside and Rights of Way Act 2000 (the 'right to roam') allows access on foot to areas of legally defined 'open country' – mountain, moor, downland, heath and registered common land. It does not allow freedom to walk everywhere. It also increases protection for Sites of Special Scientific Interest, improves wildlife enforcement legislation and allows for better management of Areas of Outstanding Natural Beauty.

How to use this book

Each of the walks in this guide are set out in a similar way. They are all introduced with a simple locator map followed by a brief description of the area, its geography and history, and some notes on things you will encounter on your walk.

Near the start of each section there is a panel of information outlining the distance of the walk, the time it is expected to take and briefly describing the path conditions or the terrain you will encounter. A suggested starting point, along with grid reference is shown, as is the nearest postcode – although in rural locations postcodes can cover a large area and are therefore only a rough guide for sat nav users. It is always sensible to take a reference map with you, and the relevant OS Explorer map is also listed.

The major part of each section is taken up with a plan for each walk and detailed point by point, description of our recommended route, along with navigational tips and points of interest.

Here is a description of the main symbols on the route maps:

Motorway	Railway station	—30m— Contour height (m)
Trunk/primary road	Bus station/stop	Walk route
Secondary road	Car park	Optional route
Tertiary road	Castle	❶ Route instruction
Residential/ unclassified road	† Church	Open land
Service road	Lighthouse	Park/sports ground
Track	★ Interesting feature	Urban area
Pedestrian/ bridleway/cycleway	*i* Tourist information	Woodland
Footway/path	Café	Nature reserve
Railway	Pub	Wetland
River/coast	Toilets	Lake

WALK 1

Hawes to Aysgill Force

The secluded valley of Sleddale offers glimpses of the area's industrial past, as well as the opportunity to spot the elusive red squirrel.

The popular market town of Hawes, whose name means a 'pass between mountains', is one of the highest in England. It lies at the heart of waterfall country, where the force of the becks that tumble down from the fells provided power to the area's mills during the Industrial Revolution. Since 1897 the town has been home to the Wensleydale Creamery, and the story of the famous cheese is told at its visitor centre. This walk also takes you through the hamlet of Gayle, where there is a fine example of a Georgian mill. Originally built as a cotton mill in about 1784, it was later converted into a saw mill and continued to operate for over a century, additionally providing electricity to the village until after the Second World War.

This strenuous circular walk follows the course of Gayle Beck, along the bottom of Sleddale, before returning to Hawes along the valley side, offering striking views of the surrounding fells, moors and crags in both directions. The natural highlight is the powerful Aysgill Force, a 50-ft (15-m) curtain of water which you will hear before you can see.

Hawes offers a selection of places to refuel after your walk. There are toilet facilities in the village and in the Dales Countryside Museum, which occupies the former railway station. As well as car parking at the National Park Centre, there is a bus link to Garsdale Railway Station.

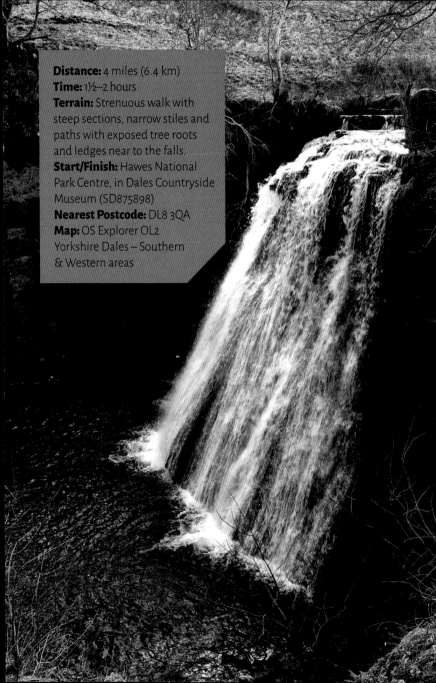

Distance: 4 miles (6.4 km)
Time: 1½–2 hours
Terrain: Strenuous walk with
steep sections, narrow stiles and
paths with exposed tree roots
and ledges near to the falls.
Start/Finish: Hawes National
Park Centre, in Dales Countryside
Museum (SD875898)
Nearest Postcode: DL8 3QA
Map: OS Explorer OL2
Yorkshire Dales – Southern
& Western areas

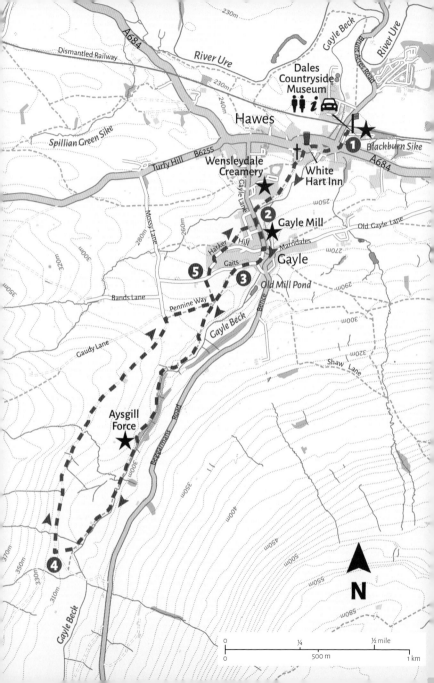

1 From the entrance to the Dales Countryside Museum, cross the road and walk into Hawes by the cobbled road. Take the footpath opposite the White Hart pub, leading up a cobbled driveway. Follow the stone-flagged path across Belah Bank to the Wensleydale Creamery.

2 Turn left and follow the road towards Gayle. Just before the bridge (from which Gayle Mill can be seen), bear right along a small lane which leads onto a cobbled footpath between quaint little cottages. Continue for a short distance on the tarmac until you see a footpath off to the left.

3 Go up the steps and follow the gentle climb across open fields to a wall. Continue through the narrow stile, following the signpost for Aysgill Force. At the next wall, cross the stile and take the path down to the left, descending the steep steps to the side of the beck. Cross another stile through the fields. The path narrows as the beck flows through a narrow-wooded gorge with steep moss and fern-covered sides. Take care approaching the falls as the path is rocky and slippery. A stone bench provides a resting point for taking in the spectacular falls. Continue forward along the beck side. Pass the concrete bridge and through more stiles. Go forward through a series of pleasant Dales meadows. After the field barn and second concrete bridge, continue forward with the beck on your left until you join a rough track.

4 Turn right onto the green lane to head back towards Hawes. Continue on the walled lane, passing farm buildings. As the track turns to tarmac road take the path on the right, signed 'Pennine Way'. Follow this through a number of fields to reach a minor tarmac road.

5 Cross the road and keep following the Pennine Way back to the Creamery. Cross the road with care and retrace your steps into Hawes town centre.

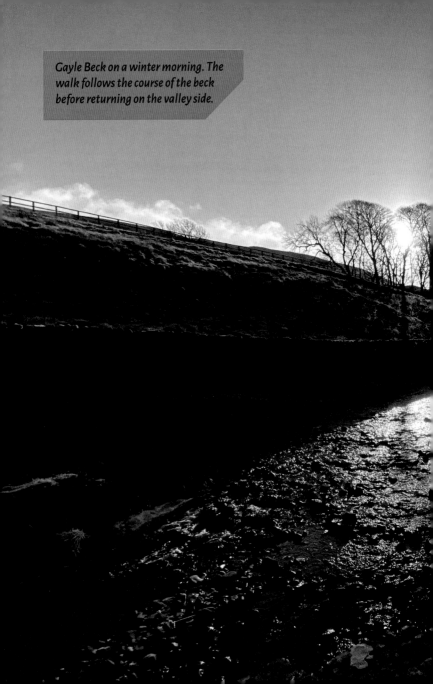

Gayle Beck on a winter morning. The walk follows the course of the beck before returning on the valley side.

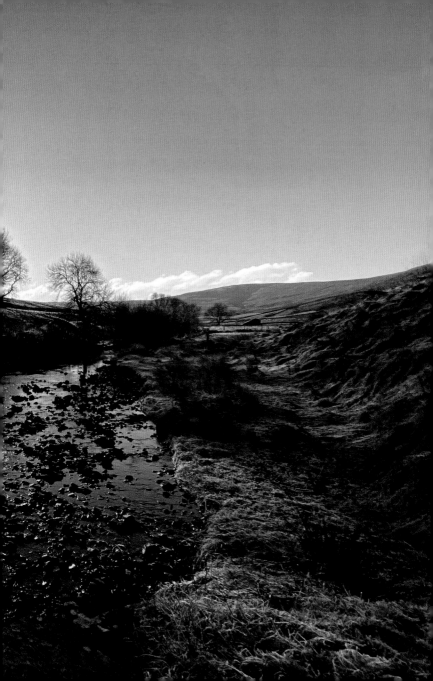

WALK 2
Malham Tarn

Take in the views of the surrounding uplands from the shores of England's highest freshwater lake.

The limestone landscape above the village of Malham contains one of only a small number of Europe's upland alkaline lakes. Malham Tarn, which is managed by the National Trust, has been designated a National Nature Reserve in recognition of the important variety of plants and wildlife that are found in and around it.

The tarn was created at the end of the last ice age, about 10,000 years ago, when a deposit of glacial moraine formed a dam across the basin. Several species of wading bird breed nearby, including oystercatchers, redshank and curlews, while on the water you may see tufted ducks, great crested grebes and teal. The freshwater molluscs that inhabit the lake are at the highest known altitude in Britain.

This circular walk begins and ends at Water Sinks, where the small stream that drains the tarn disappears below ground before re-emerging south of Malham village to form the source of the River Aire. The route takes you through woodland, across moorland and around the lake shore, and passes an isolated smelt mill chimney, a remnant of the area's nineteenth century lead mining industry.

Cafés, shops and toilets are available at nearby Malham village.

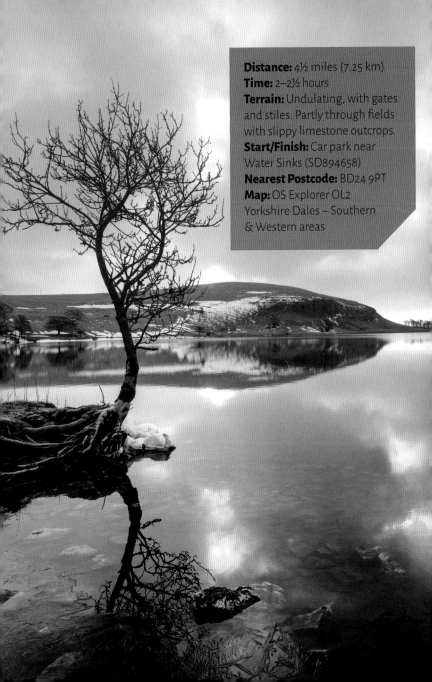

Distance: 4½ miles (7.25 km)
Time: 2–2½ hours
Terrain: Undulating, with gates and stiles. Partly through fields with slippy limestone outcrops.
Start/Finish: Car park near Water Sinks (SD894658)
Nearest Postcode: BD24 9PT
Map: OS Explorer OL2 Yorkshire Dales – Southern & Western areas

1 Leave the car park at Water Sinks, taking the Pennine Way path towards Malham Tarn. Follow the obvious grassy path next to the tarn. This path leads to a gravel track around the Tarn National Nature Reserve.

2 The track heads through pleasant woodland belonging to Tarn House and leads around the back of the house. A National Trust Information Board provides a brief history of the house and site.

3 Continue on the track and pass the house. A viewpoint to the left provides excellent views across the tarn, and a little further on there is a bird hide on the shore. Continue ahead past the cottages and look out for a track on your left. Follow this for a short while until you reach the road at a gate. You can also take an interesting diversion along the track by using the boardwalk trail.

4 Turn left and walk along the road. After 300 metres, at the first road junction, take the left fork signed to Malham. Continue along this road, passing High Trenhouse on your right. Go across the crossroads and take the gate or stile on your left to cross the open field and head towards the smelt mill chimney built in 1815.

5 Take the faint path straight ahead from the chimney, following the waymarkers for about 100 metres to the corner of the field. Continue with the wall on your left, to another wall at the brow of a hill. Go over a stile and carry on straight ahead. As the land begins to descend, bear left.

6 At the foot of the hill a track leads to a gap in the wall to your left, signed 'Public Bridleway'. Follow the path across Dean Moor until you reach the road at Water Sinks.

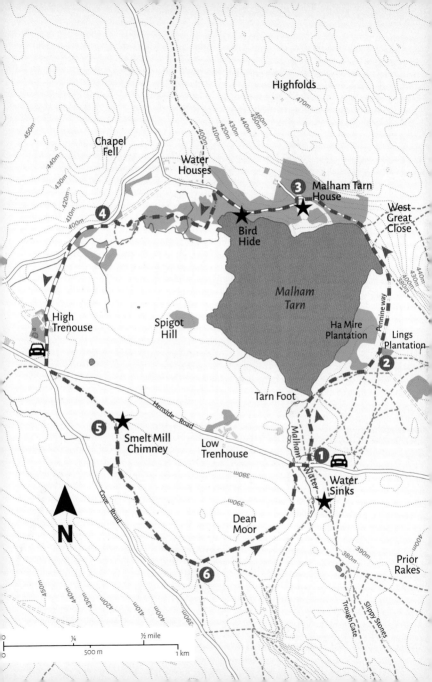

Highfolds

Chapel
Fell

Water
Houses

3 Malham Tarn
House

West
Great
Close

★
Bird
Hide

Malham
Tarn

4

High
Trenouse

Spigot
Hill

Ha Mire
Plantation

Lings
Plantation

2

Pennine way

Tarn Foot

Henside Road

5
★
Smelt Mill
Chimney

Low
Trenhouse

1

Water
Sinks

★

Cove Road

Dean
Moor

N

6

Prior
Rakes

Trough Gate

Slippy Stones

¼   ½ mile

0   500 m   1 km

WALK 3
Reeth to Healaugh

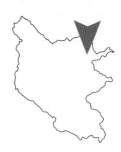

Immerse yourself in Swaledale with a walk along the wide valley floor.

The steep-sided glacial valley of Swaledale is the setting for this circular walk between the villages of Reeth and Healaugh. The area has been occupied since prehistoric times, and there is evidence of Bronze Age settlements and field systems on the valley side above Healaugh.

The attractive village of Reeth occupies a natural amphitheatre between the River Swale and the smaller Arkle Beck. It has been a market town since medieval times, and was an important centre for the woollen industry before becoming a major site for lead mining during the eighteenth and nineteenth centuries. In its heyday, Reeth was producing more than ten per cent of the country's total lead output.

This level walk skirts the steep valley side before returning along the path beside the fast-flowing River Swale, where you can look out for swallows, wagtails and dippers. The route takes you past the old Quaker school in Reeth, built in 1780, and a more modern local amenity in the form of a carpeted telephone box at Healaugh.

There are cafés, pubs, shops, toilets and a car park in Reeth, which can also be reached by bus from Richmond.

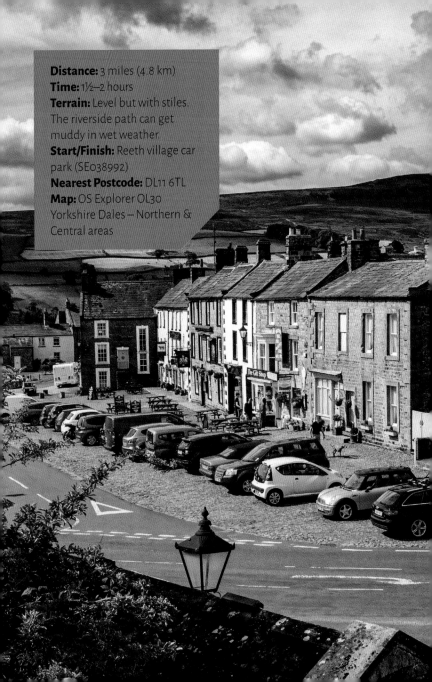

Distance: 3 miles (4.8 km)
Time: 1½–2 hours
Terrain: Level but with stiles. The riverside path can get muddy in wet weather.
Start/Finish: Reeth village car park (SE038992)
Nearest Postcode: DL11 6TL
Map: OS Explorer OL30 Yorkshire Dales — Northern & Central areas

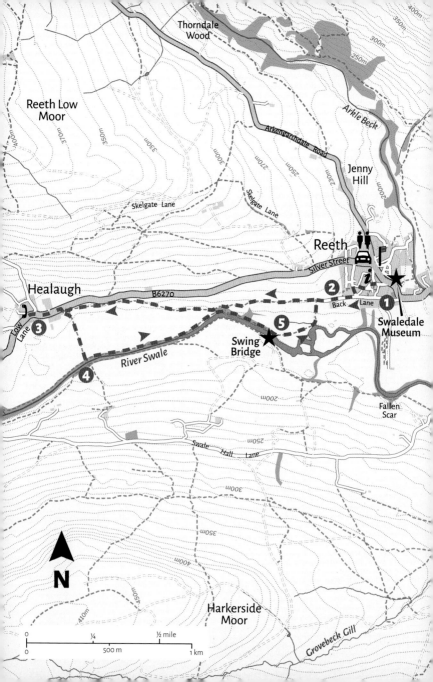

1 Starting from Reeth village green, adjacent to the car park, leave the top of the village via the narrow ginnel (passageway) next to Hudson House Information Centre, signposted to the river. After a short distance turn left and then right along narrow tarmac roads past the doctors' surgery.

2 Continue forward through to a track which has a raised footpath known as the Quaker Flags. These lead to the old Quaker school at the end of the lane. Carry on across the valley-bottom meadows, through a series of stiles and gates to the village of Healaugh, a Saxon name meaning 'high-level forest clearing'.

3 When you reach the village green, take a quick look at the well-equipped telephone box in the centre and then retrace your steps to take the footpath along the wallside that leads down to the River Swale.

4 On reaching the river turn left and head downstream, over a series of stiles to follow the pleasant riverbank to the suspension bridge, known locally as the Swing Bridge.

5 Do not cross the bridge but bear left to take the path up to a barn and walled lane. Turn right at the top of the lane to retrace your steps along the narrow tarmac road and back into the village centre.

WALK 4
Muker, Keld and the Corpse Way

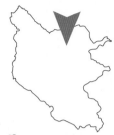

This varied walk to the head of Swaledale offers stunning views down the valley from the shoulder of Kisdon summit.

The village of Muker, whose name is from the Old Norse for 'narrow, newly cultivated field', has barely altered in the last hundred years. June is the best time to visit, when the stunning flower-rich hay meadows are in full bloom.

This circular walk follows the River Swale upstream from Muker to the peaceful village of Keld, whose population is a fraction of what it was at the peak of its lead mining activity in the late nineteenth century. Many of the houses here have had their stonework restored to its original, lighter colour.

Along the way, it is well worth the detour to visit Kisdon Force. The waterfall occupies a beautiful spot surrounded by woodland, which has been designated a Site of Special Scientific Interest (SSSI) due to the abundance of wildlife and plants.

The walk back from Keld to Muker follows part of the Corpse Way, which, until St Mary's church was built in Muker in 1580, was used by coffin bearers as they carried their dead to the nearest burial ground, ten miles (16 km) downstream at Grinton. The final part of the walk takes you over the steep shoulder of Kisdon summit and back along the Pennine Way.

Keld has a café for a half-way stop, and Muker has a pub, shop and toilets.

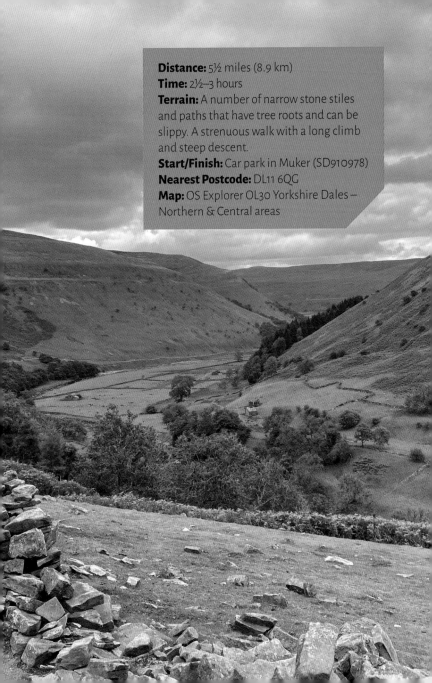

Distance: 5½ miles (8.9 km)
Time: 2½–3 hours
Terrain: A number of narrow stone stiles and paths that have tree roots and can be slippy. A strenuous walk with a long climb and steep descent.
Start/Finish: Car park in Muker (SD910978)
Nearest Postcode: DL11 6QG
Map: OS Explorer OL30 Yorkshire Dales – Northern & Central areas

1 From the car park at Muker, go up through the village and turn right by the small Post Office. Take the flagged path, signposted to Gunnerside & Keld, across the meadows until the river is reached.

2 Go through the stile, down the steps and turn left, signposted 'Footpath', and follow the waymarked route upriver passing several disused farm houses, one of which is Hartlakes, reputedly one of the most haunted places in the country. This part of the walk takes you through the old wood pasture of Muker. Look out for two pollarded alder trees on the opposite side of the river under West Arn Gill.

3 Before joining the Pennine Way National Trail, you can take a short detour along a signposted path off to the right, to Kisdon Force waterfall, a spectacular waterfall after heavy rain. Take care down the narrow slippy path. Retrace your steps and continue ahead to the hamlet of Keld.

4 Leave the village heading southeast to the main Reeth to Kirkby Stephen road. Near the War Memorial, turn left at the road junction and follow the tarmac road, signposted to Reeth & Richmond, for a quarter of a mile (400 m).

5 Take the track on the left, signposted 'Bridleway Muker', which is the old Corpse Road. Follow this track downhill and over a small footbridge. Continue ahead and start the climb onto the shoulder of Kisdon Hill. The route eventually levels out with extensive views down Swaledale, before dropping down to join the Pennine Way near Kisdon House.

6 Continue down the hill, signposted to Muker, until the village is reached. Retrace your steps back to the car park.

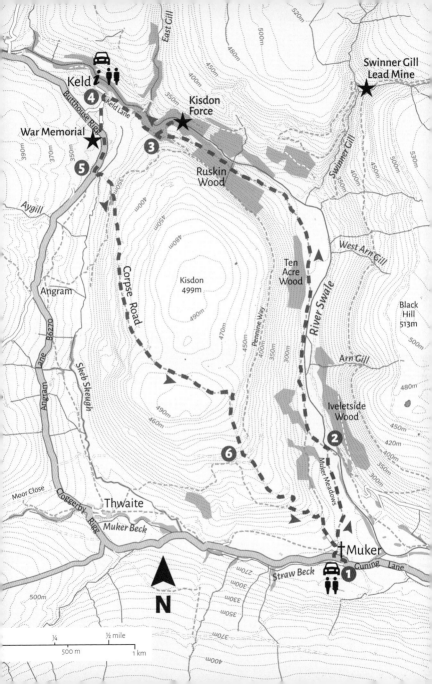

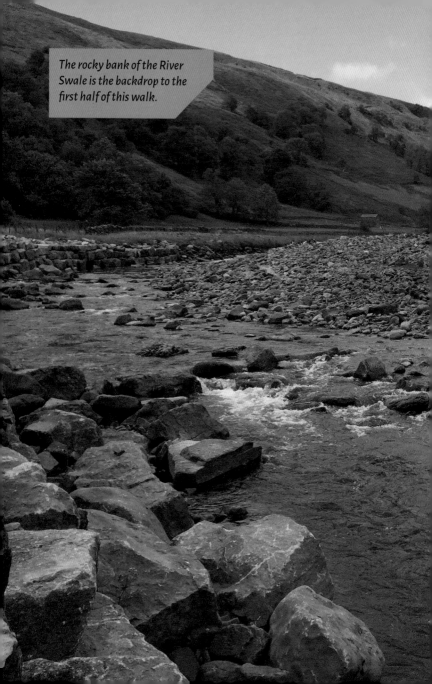

The rocky bank of the River Swale is the backdrop to the first half of this walk.

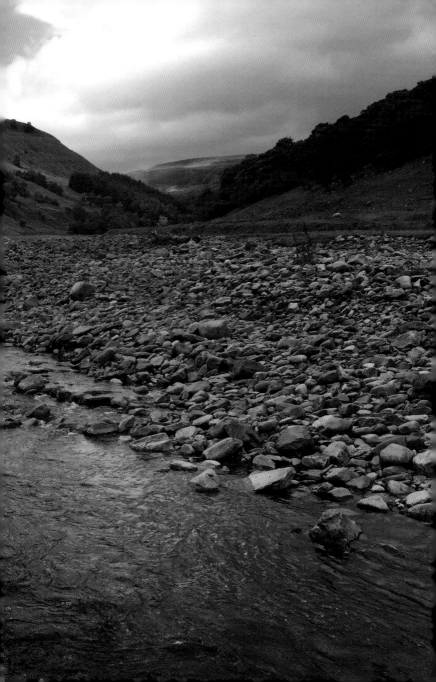

WALK 5
Smardale Gill

Industrial architecture combines with natural landforms to create a walk that is visually stunning.

In contrast to the open, rolling landscape of the surrounding countryside, Smardale Gill is a deep ravine, sliced into the hillside by Scandal Beck and filled with ancient broad-leafed woodland. During construction of the South Durham and Lancashire Union Railway, which opened in 1861, the problem of crossing the ravine was resolved by the construction of a spectacular 90-ft (27-m) fourteen-arch viaduct. The railway was used to transport coke across the Pennines to the steelworks at Barrow-in-Furness, and iron ore back to Cleveland, and was closed after a century of service.

The beautifully restored viaduct forms a striking feature across the ravine, which is managed by the Cumbria Wildlife Trust as Smardale Nature Reserve. The reserve provides protection for a wealth of plants, insects, birds and animals. The grassland that developed on the railway cuttings and embankments is particularly rich in unusual plant species, and the reserve is one of only two sites in England that is home to the Scotch argus butterfly.

Look out for roe deer, red squirrels and otters on this accessible there-and-back walk which starts and finishes at the village of Newbiggin-on-Lune, where there is a café in the garden centre. Parking is limited in the village so it is better to travel to the start by bus from Tebay or Kirkby Stephen.

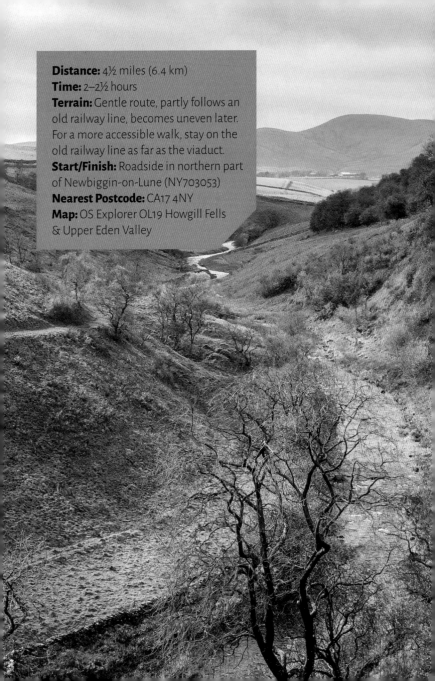

Distance: 4½ miles (6.4 km)
Time: 2–2½ hours
Terrain: Gentle route, partly follows an old railway line, becomes uneven later. For a more accessible walk, stay on the old railway line as far as the viaduct.
Start/Finish: Roadside in northern part of Newbiggin-on-Lune (NY703053)
Nearest Postcode: CA17 4NY
Map: OS Explorer OL19 Howgill Fells & Upper Eden Valley

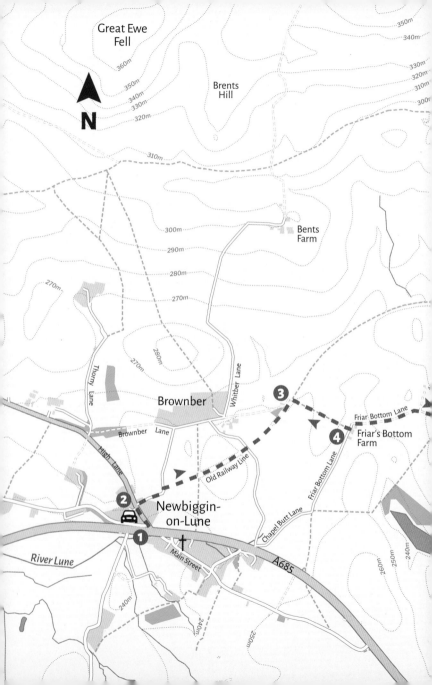

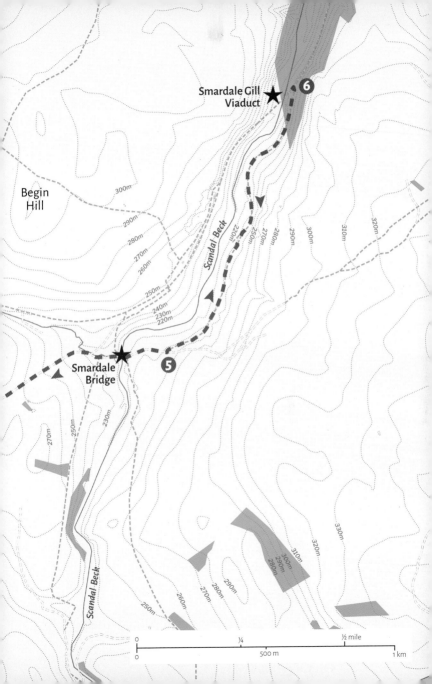

Smardale Gill
Viaduct ★ ⑥

Begin
Hill

Scandal Beck

300m
290m
280m
270m
260m
250m
240m
230m
220m

270m
260m
250m
310m
320m

★ Smardale
Bridge ⑤

Scandal Beck

270m
250m
230m

250m
260m
270m
280m
290m
300m
310m
320m
330m

280m
290m
300m

0   ¼   ½ mile
0   500 m   1 km

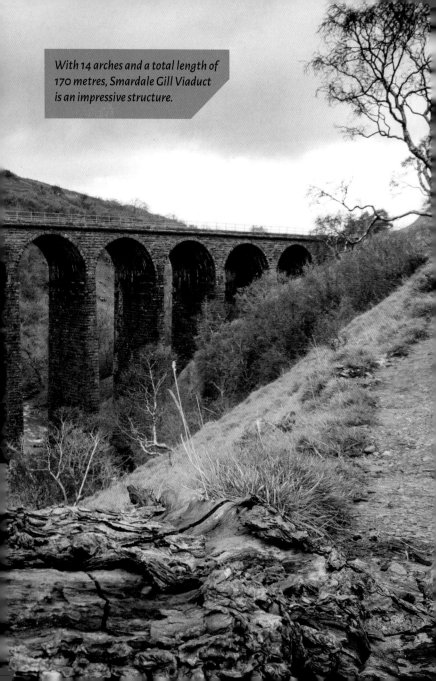

With 14 arches and a total length of 170 metres, Smardale Gill Viaduct is an impressive structure.

The village of Newbiggin-on-Lune is split by the A685 but the entirety of this walk is north of that road. Try to park in the northern part of the village by turning off the A685 in the direction of Kelleth and Great Asby. Park at the side of the road on Kelleth Lane (immediately left after you turn off the A685). If you visit the larger southern part of the village, for parking or its amenities, be careful when crossing this busy road.

1 Start the walk at the junction of High Lane and Kelleth Lane (There are two signposts here, one pointing left to 'Kelleth 2¾' and one pointing right to 'Gt Asby 7'). Follow the lane uphill towards Great Asby. After about 100 m turn right into the imposing entrance to Brownber Hall with its stone gate posts and lodge.

2 Follow the driveway for a short distance to the old railway and entrance to Smardale Nature Reserve on your right. Walk along the old railway line for nearly half a mile (600 m) until the path is crossed by a track.

3 Turn right off the old railway line and onto a bridleway which goes over a small hill to Friar's Bottom Farm.

4 At the farm, turn left onto Friar Bottom Lane and continue along the bridleway, which takes you over Smardale Bridge.

5 Follow the walled track for 150 m, and look out for a stile to your left. Go over the stile and take the path to the right through a series of disused quarries. Follow the permissive path along the valley side above Scandal Beck for three-quarters of a mile (1.2 km), and enjoy the view of the viaduct as you progress towards it.

6 Where the path meets the old railway again, at the end of the viaduct, you can climb over the stile and turn right along the railway line if you wish to go further into the nature reserve. Otherwise, turn and retrace your steps all the way back to Newbiggin-on-Lune.

WALK 6
Buckden to Cray to Hubberholme Circuit

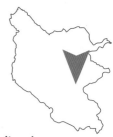

Visit three settlements on the edge of a medieval hunting forest, with breathtaking views down the glaciated valley of Wharfedale.

After forming at the tiny hamlet of Beckermonds, the young River Wharfe tumbles along Langstrothdale and passes through Hubberholme – described by the writer J. B. Priestly as the 'smallest, pleasantest place in the world' – before emerging into the wide valley of Wharfedale. This circular walk explores the area at the blunt head of Wharfedale, amid the classic Dales landscape of hay meadows, dry stone walls, glaciated valleys and steep, rugged hillsides dotted with sheep.

Starting at the village of Buckden, the route takes you up the steep, stony track of Buckden Rake to the hamlet of Cray before traversing the head of Wharfedale on the edge of Langstrothdale Chase, where it is worth taking time to enjoy the stunning views down the valley. After descending to rejoin the River Wharfe at Hubberholme, you will pass the Norman church where J. B. Priestley was laid to rest, before returning to Buckden along the valley bottom.

Buckden was established in Norman times as the administrative centre for Langstrothdale Chase, one of ten hunting forests in the Yorkshire Dales. The village was a staging post for travellers and still provides places to refuel after your walk. It can be reached by bus from Skipton.

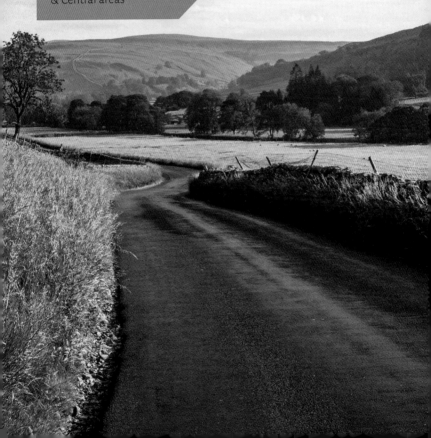

Distance: 4 miles (6.4 km)
Time: 1½–2 hours
Terrain: The steep climb out of Buckden is rough and rocky in places. The riverside path can get muddy in places.
Start/Finish: Buckden car park (SD942773)
Nearest Postcode: BD23 5JA
Map: OS Explorer OL30 Yorkshire Dales – Northern & Central areas

1 Start in the car park at Buckden and leave through the gate at the top end signposted to Buckden Pike and Cray. The stone track climbs steeply at first and can be slippery when wet. The bridleway then levels out and is flat for just over half a mile (1 km), passing through a number of gates, to a point above the small hamlet of Cray.

2 Take the footpath that drops down the hill towards The White Lion Inn, and then cross the stream via the stepping stones onto the road. The route continues around the back of the pub and follows a lovely high-level traverse above the woods through to Scar House Farm. This part of the route offers rewarding views down the classic U-shaped valley of Wharfedale, from the moorland tops down the wooded slopes to the lush valley-bottom meadows.

3 At Scar House Farm, turn left at the signpost for Hubberholme, down past the house and onto the concrete track to join the Dales Way into the village.

4 Pass the twelfth century Norman church, cross the stone arch bridge over the River Wharfe, turn left and follow the road for almost half a mile (700 m) to a gate on the left.

5 Take this footpath, signposted 'Buckden Bridge', along the pleasant riverside and meadows. Keep a lookout for kingfishers and oystercatchers, who favour this stretch of the river. Turn left when you rejoin the road to return to the village.

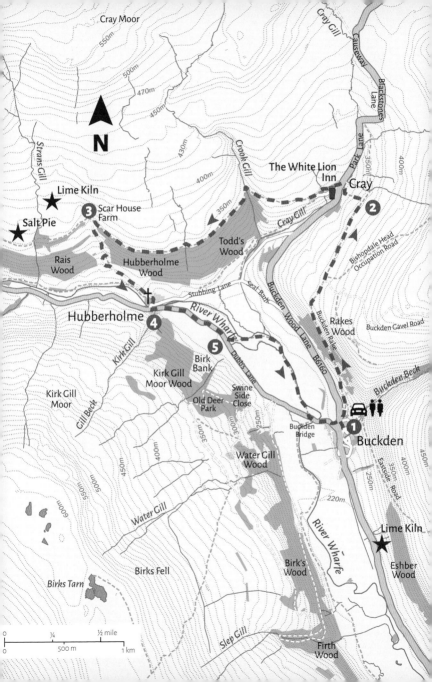

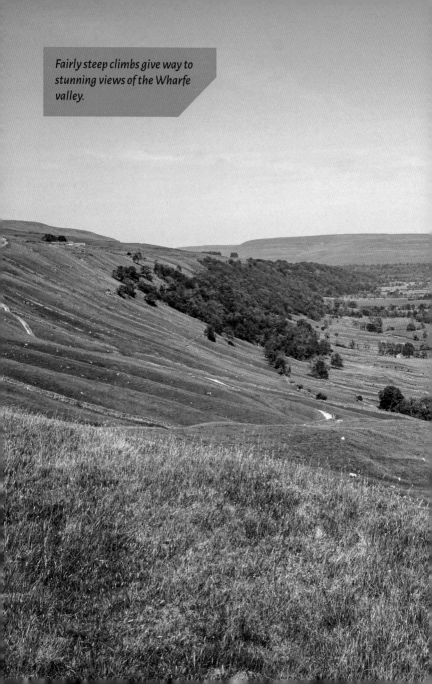

Fairly steep climbs give way to stunning views of the Wharfe valley.

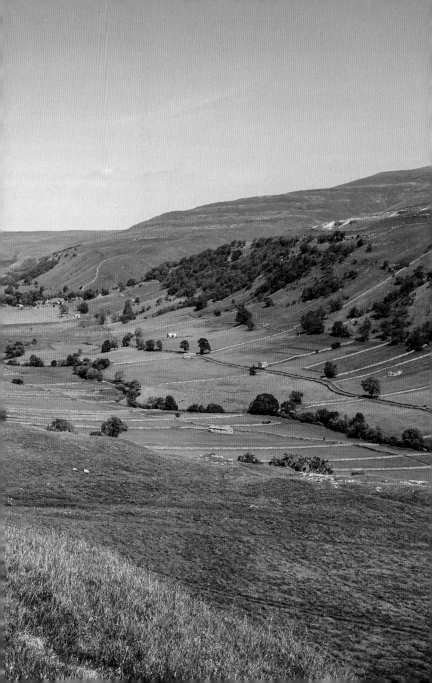

WALK 7
Orton Scar

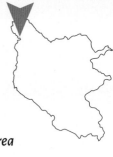

Limestone dominates the landscape here, both in the characteristic scenery of this area and in the evidence of its industrial use.

Beacon Hill Monument marks the place on the moorland above Orton Scar where a beacon was lit in 1887 to mark Queen Victoria's Golden Jubilee. The steep climb to this point is well worth it for the beautiful panoramic views of the Howgill Fells and Great Asby Scar. This limestone upland is peppered with characteristic escarpments and limestone pavements, and evidence of lime's industrial use is shown in the disused kiln that you pass on your way up the scar.

Lime has long been used as a building material, and was traditionally treated in stone kilns built close to where the stone was quarried, in order to make quicklime. Its use declined as modern materials were developed, but it is experiencing a renewed popularity in conservation projects. The sixteenth-century tower at All Saints Church in the village of Orton, where this circular walk starts and finishes, had its original lime render removed in the nineteenth century, but this was restored in 2007 in order to protect the tower from water damage. The white tower now forms a distinctive feature in the landscape and can be seen from the surrounding hills.

The village of Orton also boasts a chocolate shop, cafés and a pub. There is a limited bus service between Kendal and Ravenstonedale which passes through the village.

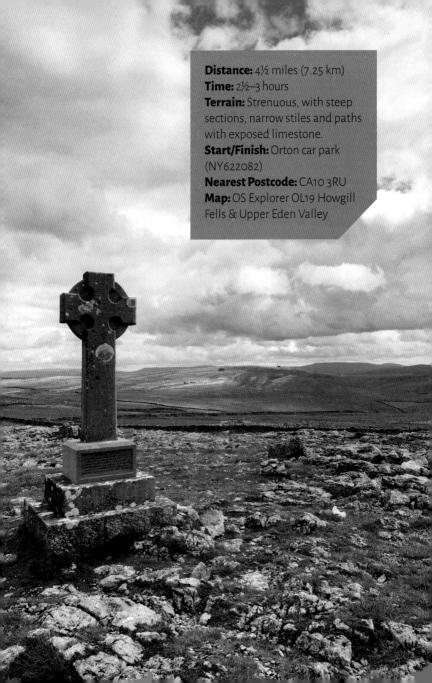

Distance: 4½ miles (7.25 km)
Time: 2½–3 hours
Terrain: Strenuous, with steep sections, narrow stiles and paths with exposed limestone.
Start/Finish: Orton car park (NY622082)
Nearest Postcode: CA10 3RU
Map: OS Explorer OL19 Howgill Fells & Upper Eden Valley

1 From the car park at Orton, take the road past All Saints Church and cross the main A6260 Appleby road with care.

2 After 100 metres turn left at a bridleway signpost. With the stream on your right-hand side, pass in front of the houses to a further signpost to the left.

3 Follow the walled lane to the gate where the bridleway opens up. Continue on the bridleway, with the stream to your right, all the way to Broadfell Farm.

4 Bear left through the farmyard. From here the route becomes steeper until you meet the road.

5 Turn right along the A6260 to where a wall runs perpendicular to the road (opposite the minor road to Crosby Ravensworth). Keeping to the wall continue until you reach Beacon Hill Monument, the highest point of the walk.

6 With the wall on your right, carry on until you reach the metal gate in the wall. Go through the gate and down the hill to pick up the bridleway. Continue for about a mile (1.7 km), until you reach a gate in the wall. From here you have a good view of the Gamelands Stone Circle.

7 Pass through the gate and follow the walled lane for a quarter of a mile (400 m). Ignoring the first footpath on the right, take the second and cross the field to a road. Turn right, pass Bland House and look out for a signpost on your right, by a large tree. Step over the stile and traverse the field to a further stile, which takes you onto a track. Cross over the track to another signpost, and cross this field to a lane. Turn right and follow the lane for 50 metres, then left over a stile at the signpost.

8 Head through the field to a narrow walled footpath. Cross the road and continue past the playing field to the centre of Orton.

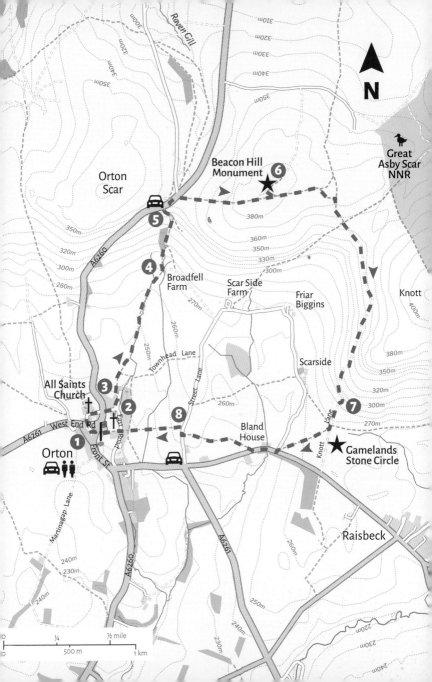

Raven Gill

300m
310m
320m
330m
340m

N

Orton
Scar

**Great
Asby Scar
NNR**

350m
350m

**Beacon Hill
Monument** ★ **6**

380m

5

350m
320m
300m
280m

360m
350m
330m
300m

Knott

4

Broadfell
Farm

270m

Scar Side
Farm

Friar
Biggins

400m

A6260

260m

250m

Townhead Lane

260m

Scarside

380m
350m
320m
300m
270m

**All Saints
Church** ✝

3

7

Street Lane

Knott Lane

2

260m

8

A6261 West End Rd

Bland
House

★ **Gamelands
Stone Circle**

1

Orton

Front St

Martinagap Lane

A6260

A6261

260m

Raisbeck

240m

230m

250m

240m

230m

220m

0   ¼   ½ mile
0   500 m   1 km

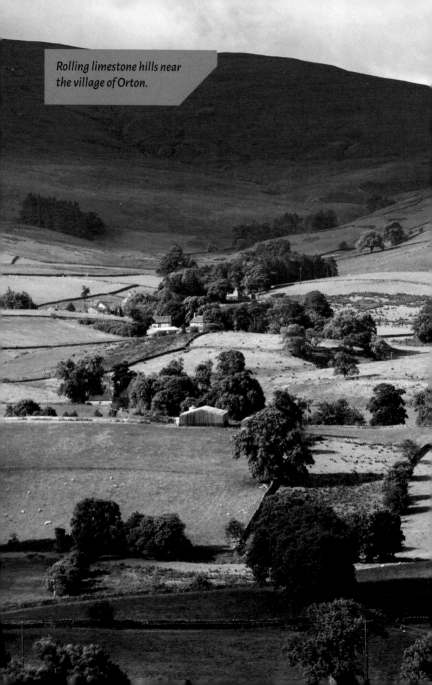

Rolling limestone hills near the village of Orton.

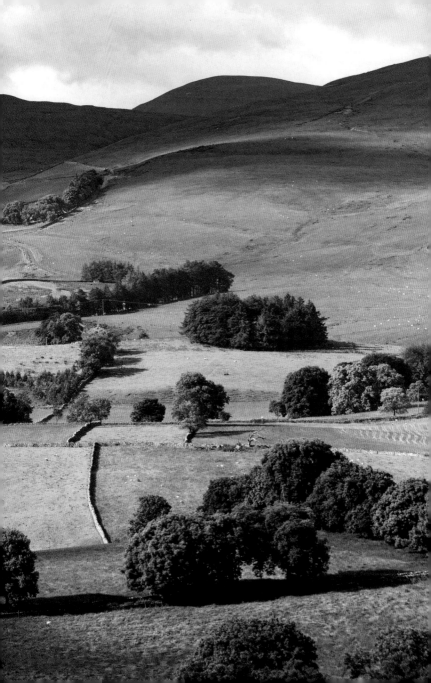

WALK 8

Stainforth and Catrigg Force

The magical waterfall of Catrigg Force offers a place of secluded contemplation in an area that has been travelled through for centuries.

The picturesque village of Stainforth takes its name from the stony ford used to cross the River Ribble between the main village and Little Stainforth on the opposite bank. By the seventeenth century, Stainforth had become a stopping off point on the packhorse route between Lancaster and York, and the ford was replaced by an arched packhorse bridge. Two centuries later, the Settle to Carlisle railway forged its way along the valley, and has been described as one of the most scenic railway lines in England.

The scenery of Ribblesdale can also be appreciated during this circular walk from Stainforth, where the magnificent panorama of the Yorkshire Three Peaks of Ingleborough, Whernside and Pen-y-ghent, which encircle the head of the valley, is a highlight of the walk. So too is the enchanting waterfall at Catrigg Force, which was a favourite of the composer Edward Elgar. A short detour from the path will take you to the waterfall, tucked away in a deep gorge, where the water of Catrigg Beck is squeezed between a narrow gap in the limestone rocks before plunging 20 ft (6 m) into the pool below.

The return to Stainforth village can be made via an impressive set of stepping stones which cross Stainforth Beck. There are toilets and a café in Stainforth, which is on the bus route between Settle and Horton in Ribblesdale.

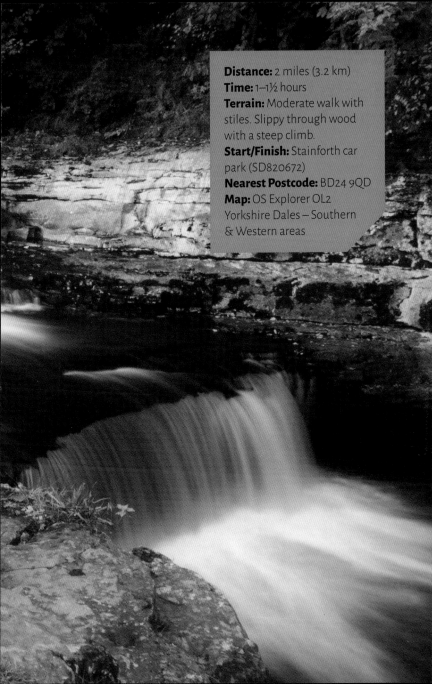

Distance: 2 miles (3.2 km)
Time: 1–1½ hours
Terrain: Moderate walk with stiles. Slippy through wood with a steep climb.
Start/Finish: Stainforth car park (SD820672)
Nearest Postcode: BD24 9QD
Map: OS Explorer OL2 Yorkshire Dales – Southern & Western areas

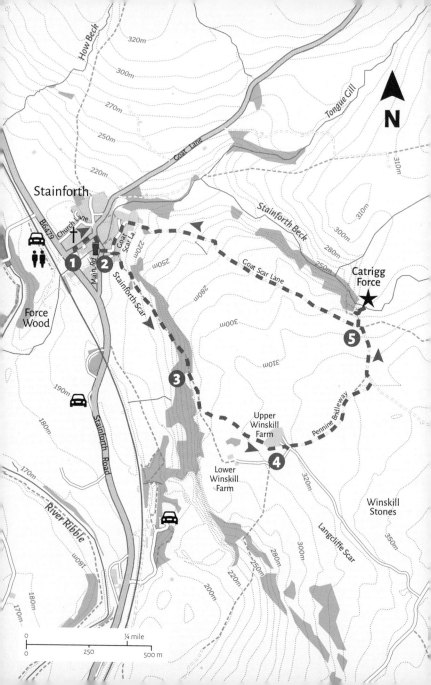

Stainforth

How Beck

Goat Lane

Tongue Gill

N

Stainforth Beck

Church Lane

BG479

Main Rd

Goat Scar La.

1

2

Goat Scar Lane

Catrigg Force

★

5

Stainforth Scar

Force Wood

Stainforth Road

3

Upper Winskill Farm

Pennine Bridleway

4

Lower Winskill Farm

Winskill Stones

Langcliffe Scar

River Ribble

0   ¼ mile
0   250   500 m

1 Leave the car park at Stainforth via the main entrance and turn right. Follow the road over the fourteenth century bridge to reach the pub on your right-hand side.

2 Take the narrow road to the left, signposted 'PBW'. Bear right and then take the footpath off to the left in between the cottages, continuing through open fields to the woodland. The path climbs up a limestone stairway through the woods above Stainforth Scar.

3 Emerging at the top of the climb, you can enjoy fine views up Ribblesdale. After leaving the woods take the left-hand path through to Upper Winskill Farm.

4 Go through the farmyard and follow the driveway. Where the main gravel track turns right, go straight ahead alongside the wall, following the bridleway signposted to Stainforth. Continue down through a gate signposted 'Pennine Bridleway Stainforth', where the Yorkshire Three Peaks will come into view: Ingleborough to the left, Pen-y-ghent to the near right and Whernside to the far right. The track leads you to the top of Goatscar Lane, a historic lane which was once part of a vital trade link between Ripon and Lancaster.

5 Go through the gate onto the lane and on the right is a path leading down to Catrigg Force waterfall – take care down the slope and near the edge. Retrace your steps to the lane and follow it down to return to Stainforth village green. Either follow the road round to the left, back to the bridge and car park, or continue ahead crossing Stainforth Beck via the stepping stones, then follow the road back to the car park.

WALK 9
Grassington Meadows

Enjoy the beautiful scenery around one of the Dales' most picturesque villages.

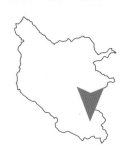

It is easy to see why Grassington is one of the most visited places in the Dales. The quaint village has changed very little over the past two hundred years, with its narrow streets and traditional stone cottages arranged around the cobbled main square. The thriving community is well known for its festivals, including the annual Dickensian Festival, which takes place in December, where shopkeepers dress in Victorian costume and market stalls and entertainers add to the festive spirit.

Situated on the bank of the River Wharfe in Upper Wharfedale, Grassington gained market town status in 1282. Lead mining began in the area in the fifteenth century, but did not develop in scale until the Industrial Revolution at the end of the eighteenth century. Tourism began at the end of the following century, when Grassington House became a boarding house, and was given a further boost by the arrival of the railway in 1902. You can learn more about rural life in Wharfedale on a visit to the Folk Museum, which is housed in two former mining cottages.

This circular walk crosses the meadows to the east of the village, and returns along the River Wharfe to the photogenic Linton Falls. Grassington has a selection of places to refuel after your walk. The village is served by buses from Skipton and Ilkley.

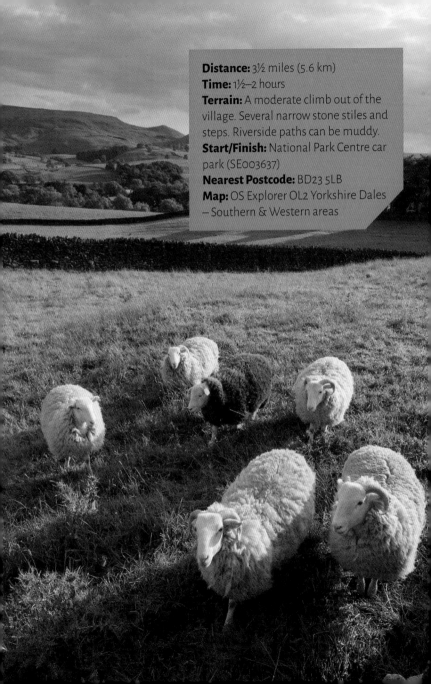

Distance: 3½ miles (5.6 km)
Time: 1½–2 hours
Terrain: A moderate climb out of the village. Several narrow stone stiles and steps. Riverside paths can be muddy.
Start/Finish: National Park Centre car park (SE003637)
Nearest Postcode: BD23 5LB
Map: OS Explorer OL2 Yorkshire Dales — Southern & Western areas

① Leave the National Park Centre car park at Grassington, heading for the village centre. Follow the road up through the village square and at the top bear right in front of the Town Hall onto Low Lane.

② After a short distance turn left onto High Lane signposted 'Hebden' and continue until you reach a footpath leading off the lane to the left.

③ The path gradually climbs through fields, crossing ancient drystone walls using stone stiles. In spring and summer birds such as lapwings and curlews can be seen and heard. Outstanding views of Barden Moor, Burnsall Fell and Cracoe war memorial can be enjoyed from here. Bear right on a footpath across the fields past the ruins of Wise House, an ancient farmstead.

④ Continue to the small coppice and turn right by the wallside, ignoring the stile. Follow the sign for the B6265 and drop down through the woods to cross the B6265 road.

⑤ Continue past Halfway House Farm to reach the River Wharfe opposite St Michael's and All Angels Church at Linton, which dates back to the twelfth century.

⑥ Ignoring the stepping stones, turn right through the gate and along the track. Continue past the hatchery until you reach the Dales Way signpost on your left. Go through the stile and down the steps to follow the riverside footpath to Linton Falls. The falls are spectacular after heavy rainfall and also at low water, when deep gouged holes can be seen. From here take the flagged narrow Sedber Lane back up to the National Park Centre.

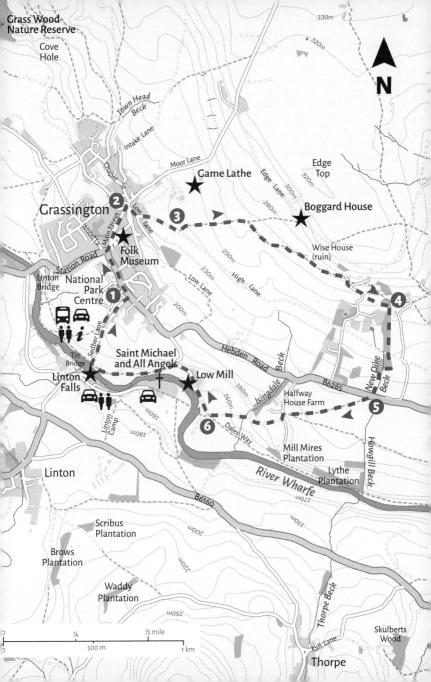

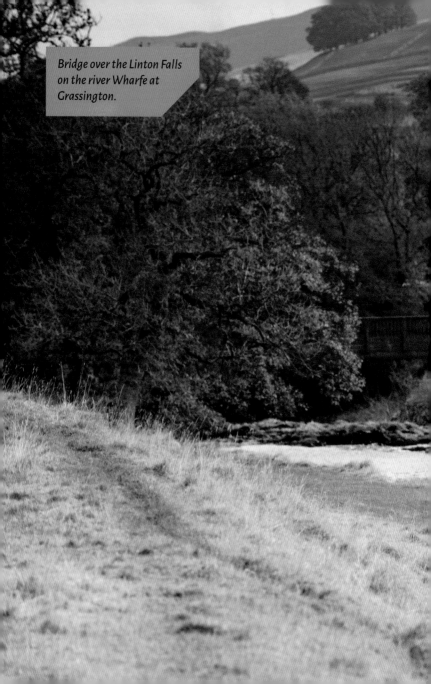

Bridge over the Linton Falls
on the river Wharfe at
Grassington.

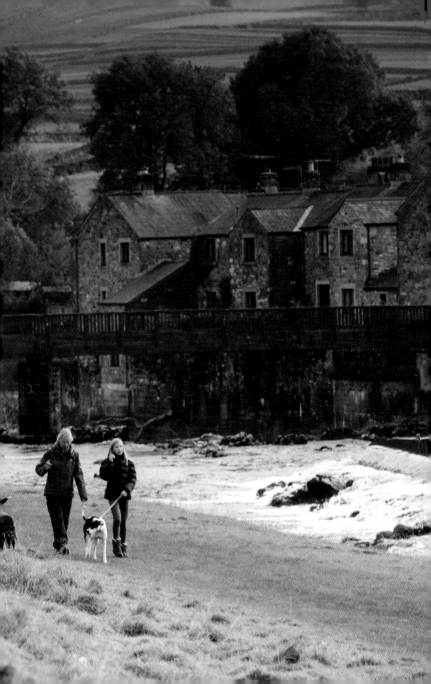

WALK 10
Reeth Low Common

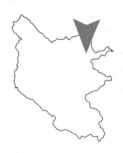

Follow in the footsteps of the lead miners in the National Park's northernmost dale.

The village of Reeth stands on the bank of Arkle Beck at the place where Arkengarthdale meets Swaledale. It is believed that lead mining may have begun in this area as far back as Roman times, though the extensive, deep-level mines were not developed until the introduction of gunpowder in the early eighteenth century. By the time the lead mining industry in Yorkshire collapsed in the early 1900s, it was possible to make the 6-mile (10-km) journey from Arkengarthdale to Gunnerside Gill in Swaledale solely via the network of underground tunnels.

On the surface, you can follow in the footsteps of the lead miners who made their way to the mines up the stone-paved lane along the side of Fremington Edge, which towers over Reeth and Arkle Beck. From here, you can see fine views of the patchwork of stone walls and field barns which characterize the area. This circular walk brings you back to Reeth along the bottom of Arkengerthdale and across the eighteenth-century road bridge.

There are shops, pubs, cafés, toilets and a car park in Reeth. The village can be reached by bus from Richmond.

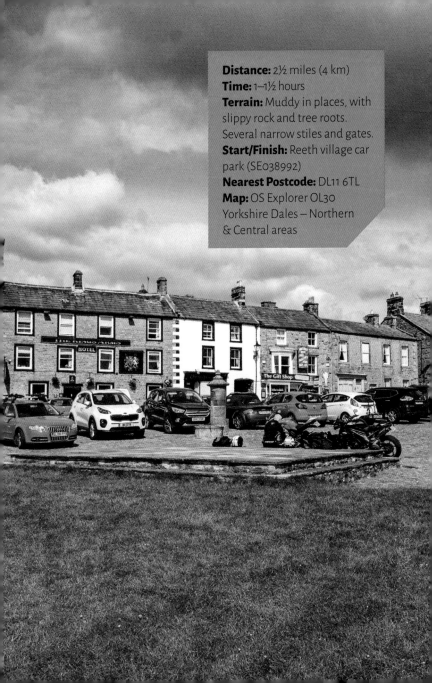

Distance: 2½ miles (4 km)
Time: 1–1½ hours
Terrain: Muddy in places, with slippy rock and tree roots. Several narrow stiles and gates.
Start/Finish: Reeth village car park (SE038992)
Nearest Postcode: DL11 6TL
Map: OS Explorer OL30 Yorkshire Dales – Northern & Central areas

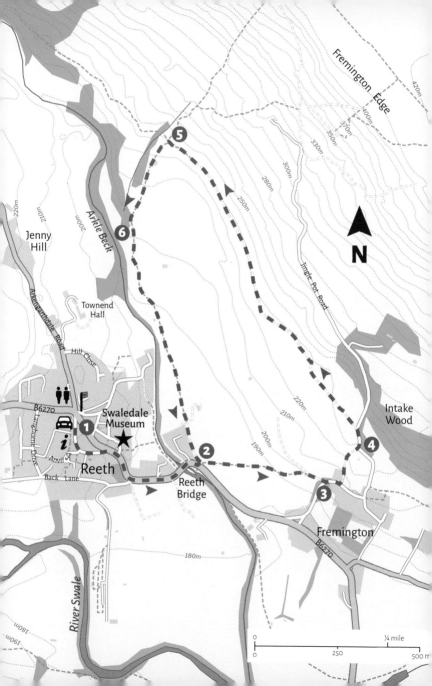

Fremington Edge

420m
400m
370m
350m
330m
300m
280m
250m

5

Arkle Beck

210m
200m

Jenny
Hill

6

Townend
Hall

Hill Close

Ingle Pot Road

220m

N

Intake
Wood

210m

B6270

Swaledale
Museum
★

Arkengarthdale Road

Langthorne Drive

Anvil Sq.

Back Lane

Reeth

1

i

2

190m

200m

Reeth
Bridge

180m

3

4

Fremington

B6270

River Swale

190m
180m

0   ¼ mile

0   250   500 m

1 Starting from the village green in Reeth adjacent to the car park, take the road down to Reeth Road Bridge, crossing with care.

2 Continuing in the same direction, take the footpath on your left across open fields towards High Fremington.

3 Bear left up a tarmac road for a short distance before turning left by the first house you reach, up onto a steep, unmarked rocky walled lane.

4 Turn left at the top and take the bridleway signposted to Arkengarthdale. Follow this pleasant grassy lane for approximately half a mile (800 m). There are fine views here of the surrounding countryside, particularly in August when the moorland tops display beautiful carpets of purple heather. Look out for traces of the old stone paved way that the miners used on their way to and from work. After a while, pass through a field gate onto the open common, and continue straight ahead to a wallside where four paths meet.

5 Take the left-hand footpath through the narrow stone stile and head down towards the field barn along the obvious well-trodden path.

6 Continue ahead on the footpath through a series of narrow stiles and gates, crossing valley-bottom meadows. To the left Fremington Edge towers above you. Traces of the old quarry workings can be seen from here. Upon reaching Reeth Road Bridge, bear right along the road and retrace your steps back to the village green.

WALK 11
Booze

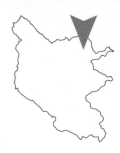

Explore the valley of Arkengarthdale, a peaceful place with a bustling past.

Despite its name, there is no pub to stop off at as you walk through the tiny hamlet of Booze. The exact origin of the name is not known, though it is thought to be Norse. The farming settlement originally developed around common land, its population expanding during the area's lead-mining days to much greater numbers than there are today. The village was hit hard by a mining disaster during the eighteenth century, when eighteen of the twenty-four men who were drowned when an underground lake was blasted, were inhabitants of Booze.

Mining in the area continued well into the nineteenth century, with slate and chert (which was used in pottery) also being extracted.

This circular walk starts and finishes in the nearby village of Langthwaite, whose bridge became familiar to many during the opening credits of the original television series of *All Creatures Great and Small*.

The walk over the side of Peat Moor Hill provides beautiful views down Arkengarthdale and Slei Gill, a steep-sided valley below Booze, before returning alongside Arkle Beck through a pretty wood, which is carpeted with bluebells in the spring.

There are pubs and toilets in Langthwaite, and a small car park on the main road just south of the village.

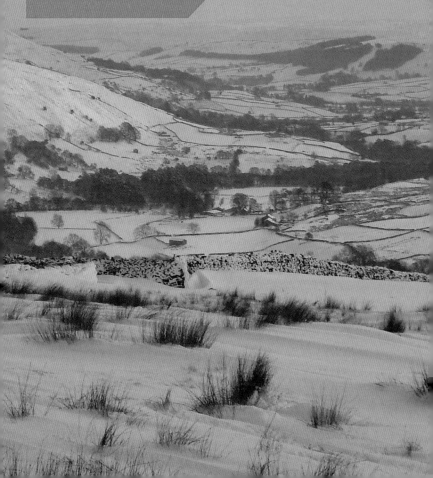

Distance: 3¼ miles (5.2 km)
Time: 1½–2 hours
Terrain: Grassy paths with some steepish slopes, gates and stiles.
Start/Finish: Small car park south of Langthwaite (NZ005023)
Nearest Postcode: DL11 6RD
Maps: OS Explorer OL30 Yorkshire Dales – Northern & Central areas

1 From the car park south of Langthwaite, walk into the village and turn right to cross the hump-backed bridge over Arkle Beck. Cross the square with the Red Lion Inn to one side and fork left on an upward-slanting woodland path for about half a mile (800 m) until you reach a path off to the right.

2 Turn right and climb to open fields above woodland, passing a ruined farmhouse. Turn right through a wicket gate marked by a finger post. Climb slightly right and uphill along the path marked by posts for a quarter of a mile (400 m).

3 At the top of the rocky field, go through a gate and follow a track to the right, across the heather moor for nearly half a mile (640 m).

4 On reaching the boundary wall, follow it bearing right as far as a barn. Climb a stile to its right and follow the sunken field path that zigzags downhill.

5 Turn left along the lane into the farm hamlet of Booze.

6 Turn right through the stockyard at Town Farm. There is no path but go down the middle of two adjacent fields towards the valley bottom.

7 Bear right along a grassy path above the stream then right again into the main valley.

8 Do not cross the footbridge on your left but continue upstream along the riverside track which takes you back to Langthwaite.

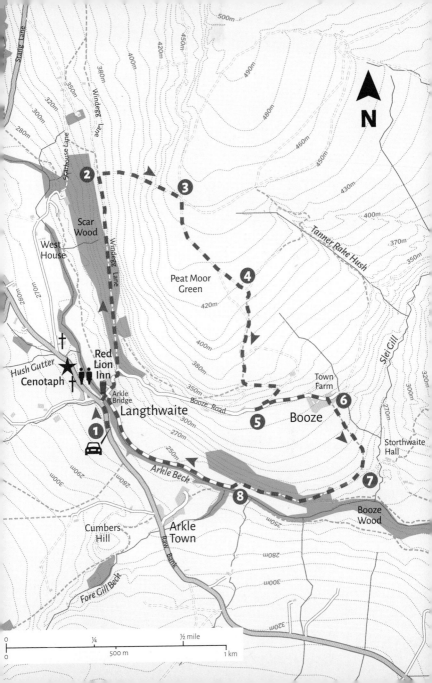

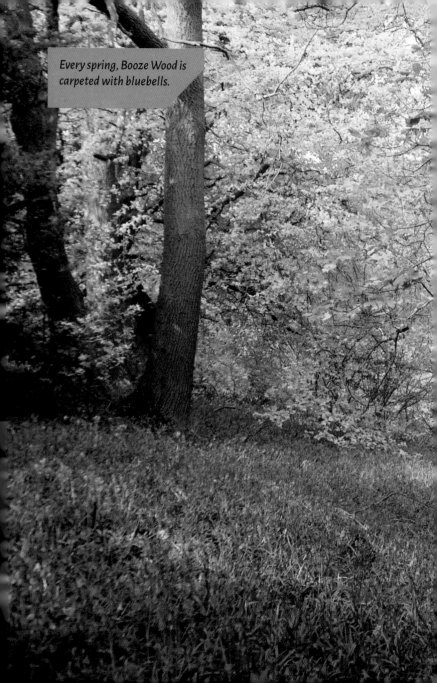

Every spring, Booze Wood is carpeted with bluebells.

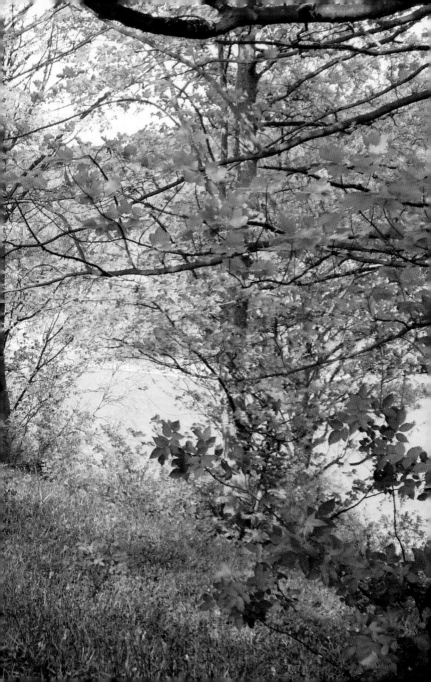

WALK 12
Semerwater

A gentle walk along a fascinating valley that is rich in archeological and natural history.

Bainbridge is the starting point for this circular walk that takes you up the River Bain which, at just over 2 miles (3.2 km) long, is thought to be England's shortest named river. It drains from the northern end of Semerwater, where the dramatic scene across the lake was painted by the landscape artist J. M. W. Turner in about 1820.

Semerwater is one of only two natural lakes in the Yorkshire Dales and, like Malham Tarn, was formed at the end of the last ice age. Bronze Age spears used to hunt deer and wild horses that came to drink from the lake have been found on its shores. It is now a haven for wildlife, and the site of a nature reserve which hosts a variety of water birds and waders, along with wild-flowers such as devil's-bit scabious. If you're lucky, you may also see roe deer in the autumn.

As you return to Bainbridge, you will pass the remains of a Roman fort built on the summit of Brough Hill, overlooking the confluence of the rivers Ure and Bain. The fort was an important military centre for over 300 years and controlled the principal pass through the Pennines.

Bainbridge has a pub, shop, café and car park. The village is on the bus route between Leyburn and Gayle.

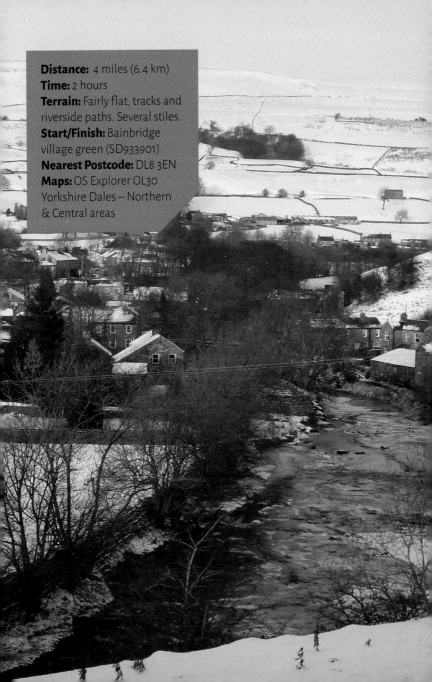

Distance: 4 miles (6.4 km)
Time: 2 hours
Terrain: Fairly flat, tracks and riverside paths. Several stiles.
Start/Finish: Bainbridge village green (SD933901)
Nearest Postcode: DL8 3EN
Maps: OS Explorer OL30 Yorkshire Dales – Northern & Central areas

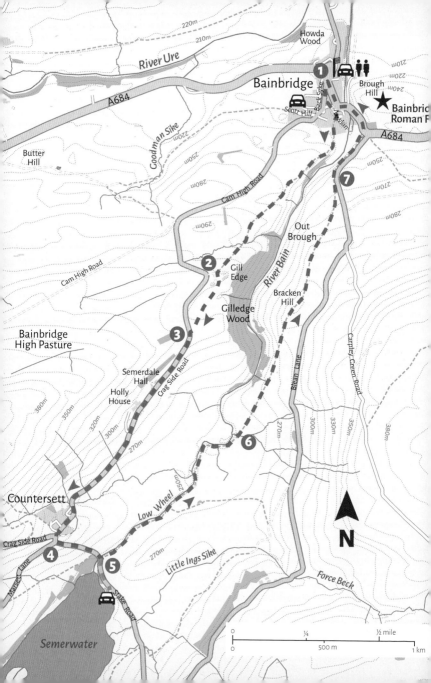

1 Follow the 'No through road' away from Bainbridge village green to the south, past Dame's School cottage and then along a private drive marked with a footpath sign. Climb away from the house, to the right and into open fields, passing the remains of the Roman fort in about ¼ mile (400 m).

2 Keep to the right of the large house at Gill Edge, as indicated by signposts and then cross the dip of the next field.

3 Go through the stile to the right of the barn and turn left along Crag Side Road.

4 Bear left through the small hamlet of Countersett and follow the road downhill to Semerwater. A short detour along the road will take you to the lake shore, where you will see a large boulder called the Carlow Stone. Return to the triple-arched Semer Water Bridge, but don't cross it.

5 Go through the narrow stile on the right next to the bridge and follow the riverside path signposted to Bainbridge. Keep to the riverbank for ¾ mile (1.2 km).

6 Climb a ladder stile and bear right uphill. Keep well to the left of the road and follow occasional waymark posts for a little over a mile (1.6 km).

7 Join the side road and follow it down to the main road. Turn left and pass the site of the Roman fort as you walk back into Bainbridge.

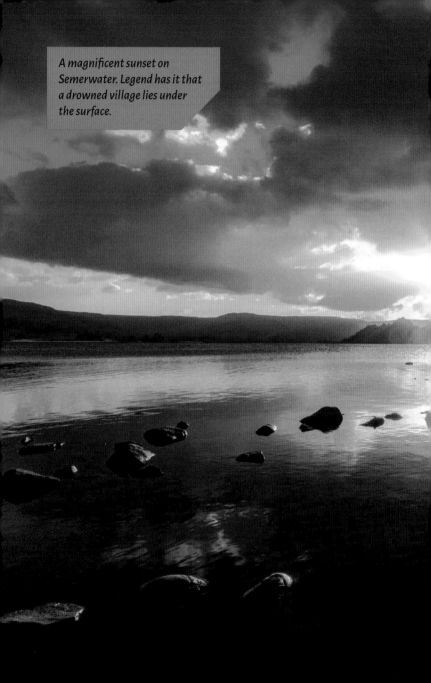

A magnificent sunset on Semerwater. Legend has it that a drowned village lies under the surface.

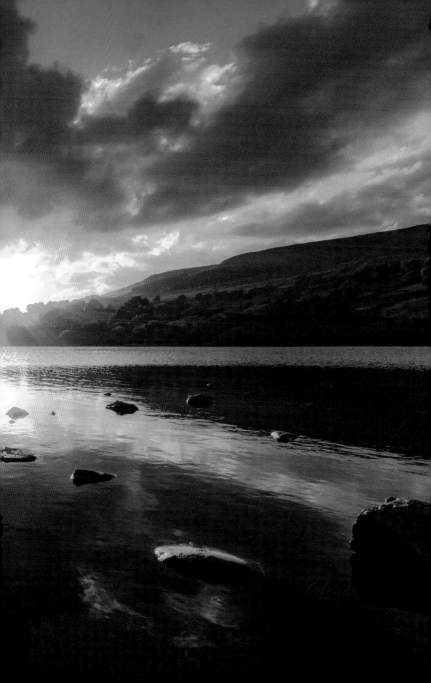

WALK 13
Hell Gill

Hell Gill Beck creates dramatic features on this walk along a little-known border valley.

This circular walk starts at Lunds, a district of small, scattered farms at the head of Wensleydale. As you climb Lunds Fell you will see the redundant church that was built as a chapel of ease in the mid-eighteenth century. Chapels like this served remote parts of parishes, where the residents lived too far from the main parish church to attend. A level path along the fellside then takes you to the bridge over Hell Gill, a quarter-mile (400-m) long, narrow, vertical-sided gorge known as a slot canyon, which has been sliced through the limestone by Hell Gill Beck. Further downstream you will pass the small but beautiful waterfall of Hellgill Force, before you cross Aisgill Moor.

Aisgill Moor is a high, flat moor forming the watershed between the River Ure, which flows south then eastward to ultimately drain into the North Sea, and the River Eden, which flows north and westward to the Solway Firth. The moor is the highest point on the Settle to Carlisle railway, and if you are lucky you might see a steam train passing through this little-known valley, on the boundary of North Yorkshire and Westmorland and Furness.

There are no facilities along this walk. The nearest pub is a mile (1.6 km) south of Lunds.

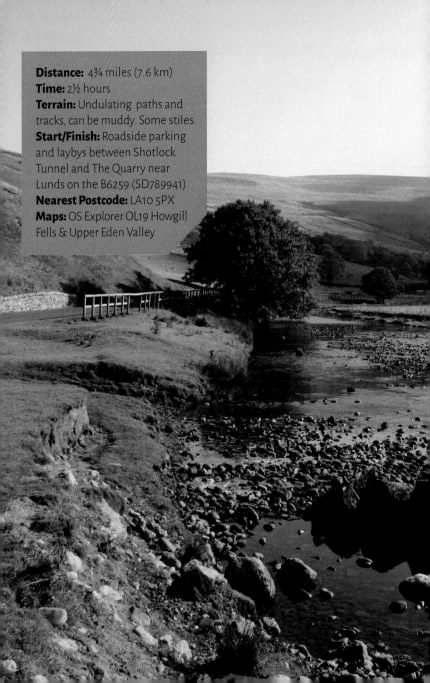

Distance: 4¾ miles (7.6 km)
Time: 2½ hours
Terrain: Undulating paths and tracks, can be muddy. Some stiles.
Start/Finish: Roadside parking and laybys between Shotlock Tunnel and The Quarry near Lunds on the B6259 (SD789941)
Nearest Postcode: LA10 5PX
Maps: OS Explorer OL19 Howgill Fells & Upper Eden Valley

1 From the roadside parking place on the B6259 at Lunds, walk down the road, away from the plantation to a footpath sign near the quarry. Turn left across a rough field and follow a waymarked footpath through the wood. Turn right along the forest drive up to Lunds Church.

2 Follow a signposted footpath to Shaws, the tree-sheltered white house high on the hillside.

3 Turn left over the bridge then bear right above the house. Follow a faint path up the hillside for another 100 metres or so.

4 Climb a stone stile and turn left along to follow the level moorland track for 1½ miles (2.4 km), taking you past a viewpoint close to the head of the River Ure and on to Hell Gill Bridge.

5 Cross the bridge, peering over the edge to see the slot canyon below, then turn left down the farm track. Cross the railway bridge and continue to the road, passing Hellgill Force.

6 Cross the road. Follow a signposted path up to a gate. There is no path, so follow the moorland boundary wall along its right side for about a mile (1.6 km).

7 Go half-right through the abandoned farmyard and, still following the boundary wall, aim for the gate in the corner of the next field.

8 Keep level across the pathless moor for about ¼ mile (400 m). Then descend gradually to the left, towards the railway tunnel.

9 Keep above the portal of Shotlock Tunnel. Go through the gate and turn right along the road and back to the start.

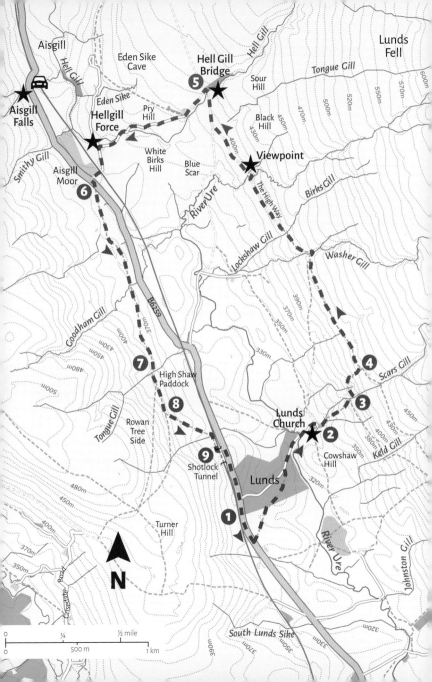

Aisgill

Hell Gill

Lunds Fell

Eden Sike Cave

Hell Gill Bridge

Tongue Gill

Sour Hill

5

Eden Sike

Pry Hill

Black Hill

Aisgill Falls

Hellgill Force

Viewpoint

Smithy Gill

White Birks Hill

Blue Scar

River Ure

Aisgill Moor

6

The High Way

Birks Gill

Lockshaw Gill

Washer Gill

B6259

Goodham Gill

4

Scars Gill

High Shaw Paddock

7

8

Lunds Church

2

Cowshaw Hill

Keld Gill

Tongue Gill

Rowan Tree Side

9

Shotlock Tunnel

Lunds

River Ure

1

Turner Hill

Johnston Gill

South Lunds Sike

N

0 ¼ ½ mile

0 500 m 1 km

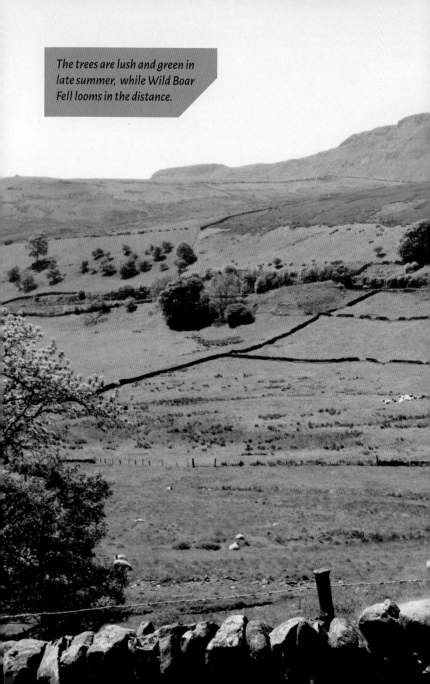

The trees are lush and green in late summer, while Wild Boar Fell looms in the distance.

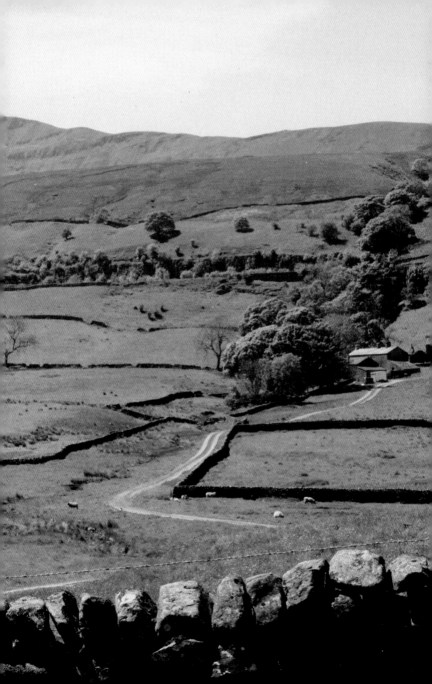

WALK 14
Winder

The summit of Winder offers a stunning panorama of the Yorkshire Dales, the Lake District hills, and the Lune Valley stretching down to Morecambe Bay.

To the locals, Winder (which rhymes with cinder) is known simply as 'The Fell'. It is an outlier of the glorious rolling hills known as the Howgill Fells, whose southern half occupies the northwestern corner of the National Park. The pupils of Sedbergh School sing of their love for Winder and the friendly protection it offers by sheltering their town from the north winds.

The landscape of the Howgill Fells differs from the limestone scenery that characterizes the rest of the Yorkshire Dales because the underlying rock consists of slates and gritstones, which were laid down millions of years before the limestone to the east. The fells have a rounded, grassy form, and from the summit of Winder it is not difficult to see why they have been likened to a huddle of squatting elephants.

The town of Sedbergh is the starting point for this circular walk. Sitting at the foot of the Howgills, on the north bank of the River Rawthey, the town's history dates back to at least the Norman times, when the motte and bailey castle of Castlehaw Tower was built. The town prospered as a result of farming and the woollen garments industry.

Choose a clear day for this walk across open country. Sedbergh offers plenty of facilities for before and after the walk, and transport links by train and bus.

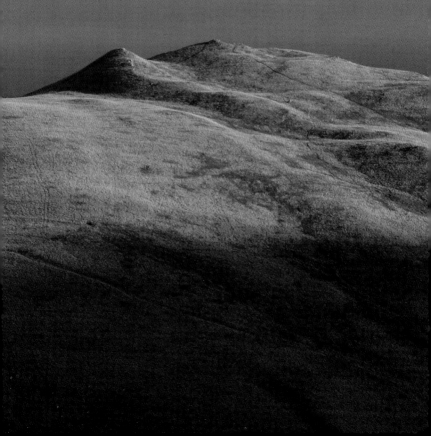

Distance: 4¾ miles (7.6 km)
Time: 2½ hours
Terrain: Strenuous walk on grassy unmarked paths with an ascent of over 300 m.
Start/Finish: Loftus Hill car park, Sedbergh (SD657919)
Nearest Postcode: LA10 5RX
Maps: OS Explorer OL19 Howgill Fells & Upper Eden Valley

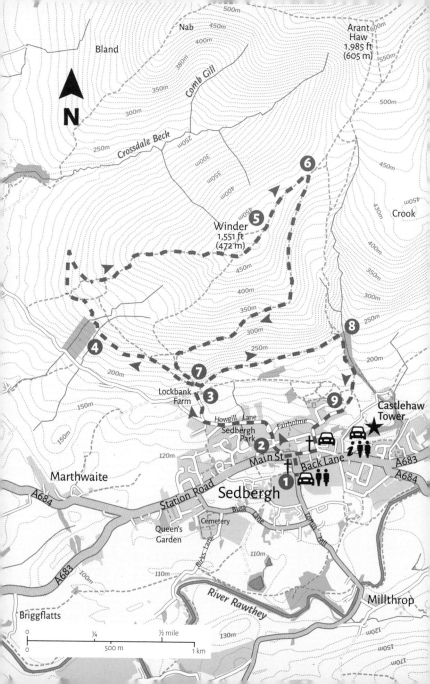

1 From the Loftus Hill car park in Sedbergh, turn right and then left along the High Street.

2 Turn right and follow Howgill Lane to the end of the 30 mph limit. Then turn right on a path marked 'To the Fell'. Walk up to Lockbank Farm.

3 Go half-right through the farmyard, then left by the grassy path alongside the boundary wall.

4 Follow the wall above a pinewood and turn right on a steeply inclined path towards the rounded summit of Winder.

5 Continue ahead and downhill along the grassy ridge to a broad col.

6 Take a sharp right-hand turn and go downhill, following a well-made path for a further mile (1.6 km).

7 Go downhill as far as the intake gate at Lockbank Farm. Turn left away from the farm, again following the fell boundary for half a mile (800 m).

8 Turn right through a kissing gate and walk downhill to the right of a shaley wooded gorge.

9 Follow the farm lane to the right, into the outskirts of Sedbergh. The church and central car parks are on the right of the town centre.

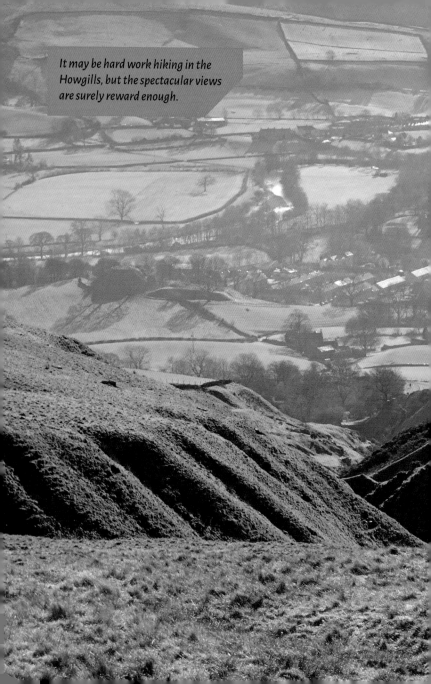

It may be hard work hiking in the Howgills, but the spectacular views are surely reward enough.

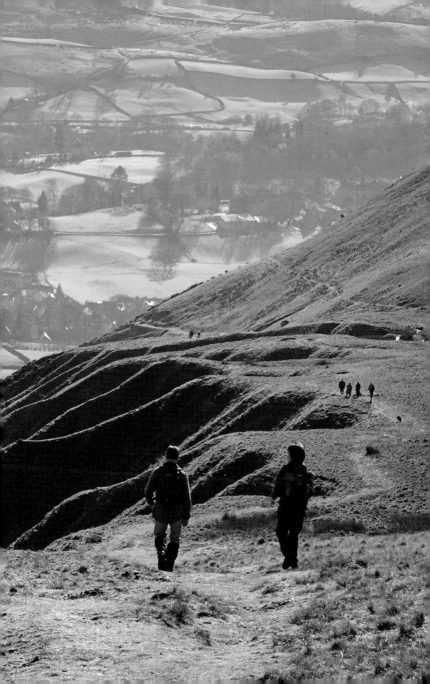

WALK 15
Middleham

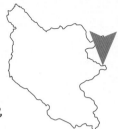

A walk at the heart of horse racing country, where King Richard III trained for battle.

The imposing ruins of the castle at Middleham dominate the historic market town which lies to the east of the National Park in Wensleydale. The great tower was begun in the late twelfth century, and successive additions were made until, by the mid-fifteenth century, the castle had become a fortified palace and a fitting residence for the powerful Earls of Westmoreland and of Warwick. In 1465, the 13-year-old Duke of Gloucester came to Middleham to spend three years learning knighthood skills from his cousin the Earl of Warwick. The Duke was later crowned Richard III, and continued to spend time at the castle during his short and turbulent reign, which ended with his defeat in the Wars of the Roses.

For over two centuries the moorland surrounding Middleham has been used for training racehorses and the town is now the centre of a thoroughbred breeding area which has earned it the nickname the 'Newmarket of the North'.

This strenuous circular walk takes you from the centre of the town and over the Low Moor past William's Hill, the remains of an earlier castle, before descending to the wooded valley of the River Cover. You will walk past the pretty arched stone bridge of Hullo Bridge before returning past Pinker's Pond to Middleham, where there are pubs, cafés, shops and parking.

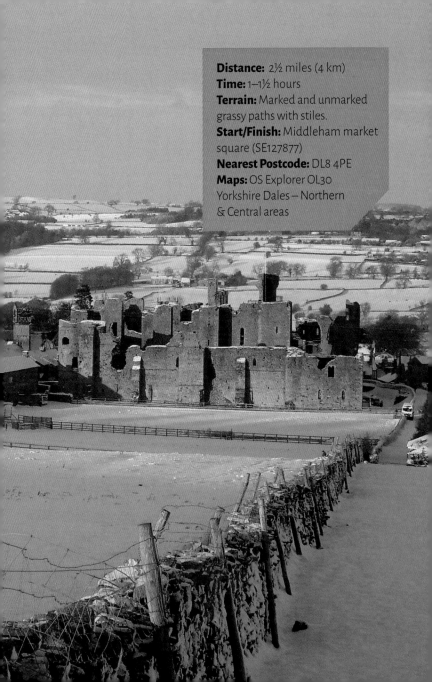

Distance: 2½ miles (4 km)
Time: 1–1½ hours
Terrain: Marked and unmarked grassy paths with stiles.
Start/Finish: Middleham market square (SE127877)
Nearest Postcode: DL8 4PE
Maps: OS Explorer OL30 Yorkshire Dales – Northern & Central areas

1 From the market square in Middleham, follow the lane on the left of the castle southwards into open fields. Keep the boundary wall on your right beyond the house at the lane end, and climb up and over the shoulder of Middleham Low Moor, passing the earthwork remains of the early castle of William's Hill to your right.

2 Bear right towards the trees lining deep-cut Coverdale. Follow the woodland boundary fence as far as a clump of pine trees.

3 Climb two stiles at the edge of the wood. Bear half-left, downhill across the next field.

4 Walk down to the old but well-built Hullo Bridge. Do not cross the river but turn right, away from the bridge and climb along a well-defined cart track for half a mile (800 m).

5 Follow the track up to the unfenced road. Cross the road and follow red posts up to walk on the pathless grassy swathe of Middleham Moor.

6 Cross the moor, then bear right, back towards the road. Turn left onto the road, which takes you back into Middleham.

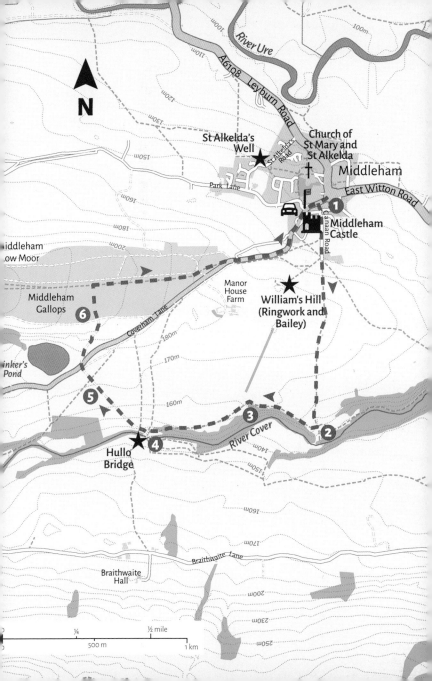

River Ure

A6108 Leyburn Road

100m

110m

120m

130m

150m

160m

St Alkelda's Well

St Alkelda Road

Park Lane

Church of St Mary and St Alkelda

Middleham

East Witton Road

1

Canaan Road

Middleham Castle

...iddleham ...ow Moor

200m

Middleham Gallops

6

Coverham Lane

Manor House Farm

William's Hill (Ringwork and Bailey)

180m

170m

...inker's Pond

160m

5

3

River Cover

2

Hullo Bridge

4

140m

150m

160m

Braithwaite Lane

170m

Braithwaite Hall

200m

230m

250m

N

¼   ½ mile

500 m   1 km

Middleham market square marks the start and end point of this lovely little walk.

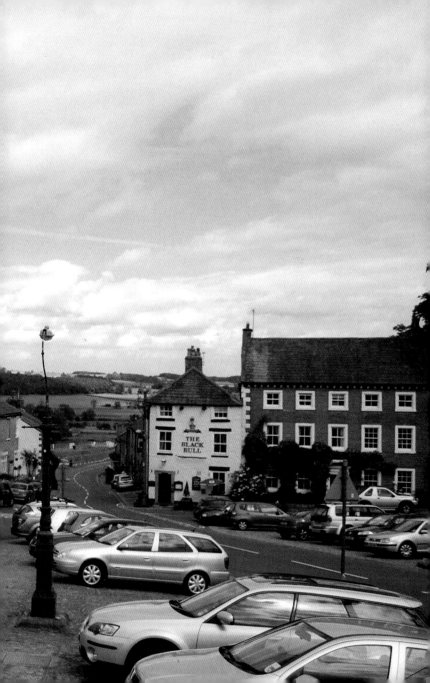

WALK 16
Kettlewell and Starbotton

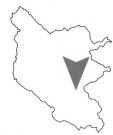

Enjoy a lovely riverside walk along the Wharfe, whose name is from the Norse for 'winding river'.

The two picturesque Dales villages of Kettlewell and Starbotton sit on the northeast bank of the River Wharfe in Upper Wharfedale. This area has a long history of human occupation and both villages were listed in the Domesday Book. Many of the buildings in the villages date back to the late seventeenth century and were built to replace those that had been destroyed by a flash flood which swept through this part of Wharfedale in June 1686 following heavy rainfall on the surrounding fellsides.

Around both villages there is evidence of a long history of farming, as well as the remains of the lead mining industry that was so important in this part of Yorkshire during the eighteenth and nineteenth centuries.

It is a pleasant, gentle walk between the two villages, and particularly pretty in spring and summer. This route takes you from Kettlewell, along a centuries-old field path that contours the valley side at Cam Pasture, to Starbotton. The return route brings you back along the riverside following part of the Dales Way, an 80-mile long-distance footpath linking Bowness-on-Windermere in Westmorland and Furness with Ilkley in West Yorkshire.

There are pubs in both villages, plus toilets and a shop in Kettlewell, which is connected by bus to Skipton and Buckden.

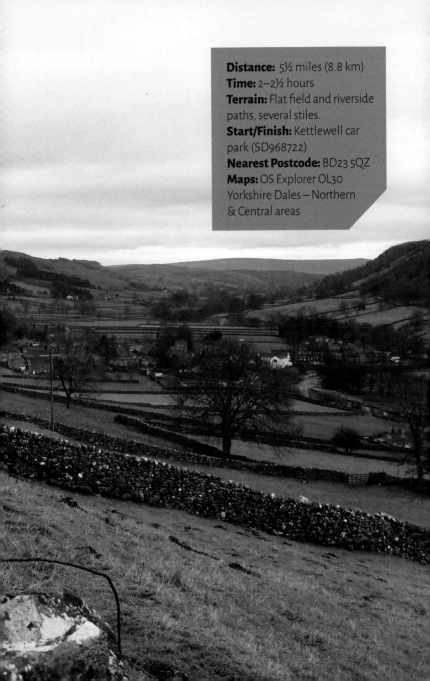

Distance: 5½ miles (8.8 km)
Time: 2–2½ hours
Terrain: Flat field and riverside paths, several stiles.
Start/Finish: Kettlewell car park (SD968722)
Nearest Postcode: BD23 5QZ
Maps: OS Explorer OL30 Yorkshire Dales – Northern & Central areas

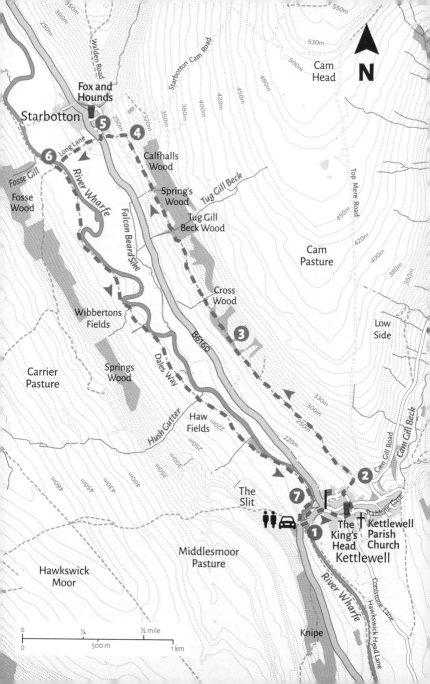

1 From the car park at Kettlewell, walk towards the church. Turn left at The King's Head for about 20 metres, passing the youth hostel. Turn right along a grassy lane.

2 Climb the stile at the lane head and turn left to follow the boundary wall.

3 Cross all intervening boundary walls by their stiles for a total of 1¾ miles (2.8 km).

4 Go left through a metal gate. Then turn half-right, to walk downhill towards Starbotton village.

5 To visit the village, turn right along the main road, otherwise cross the road and follow the walled lane down to the river.

6 Cross the footbridge over the River Wharfe and turn left to join the route of the Dales Way, following the river downstream for 2 miles (3.2 km) through a series of meadows. The path above the river meanders so always use stiles to keep to the correct route.

7 Follow the curve of the riverbank below Kettlewell. Turn left over the double road bridge to return to the village.

WALK 17
Simon's Seat

Spectacular grandstand views are the reward for the steep climb to this summit.

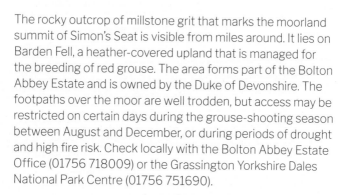

The rocky outcrop of millstone grit that marks the moorland summit of Simon's Seat is visible from miles around. It lies on Barden Fell, a heather-covered upland that is managed for the breeding of red grouse. The area forms part of the Bolton Abbey Estate and is owned by the Duke of Devonshire. The footpaths over the moor are well trodden, but access may be restricted on certain days during the grouse-shooting season between August and December, or during periods of drought and high fire risk. Check locally with the Bolton Abbey Estate Office (01756 718009) or the Grassington Yorkshire Dales National Park Centre (01756 751690).

Dogs are not allowed on the moor at any time.

There are various theories about the origin of the summit's name: one that it was named after a baby found by a shepherd boy, while another claims that it is a Druid name relating to the first-century religious figure Simon Magus.

This circular walk offers an alternative route up Simon's Seat to the more popular path from Bolton Abbey, and starts at the hamlet of Howgill. All facilities can be found in the nearby village of Appletreewick, which is served by buses from Ilkley.

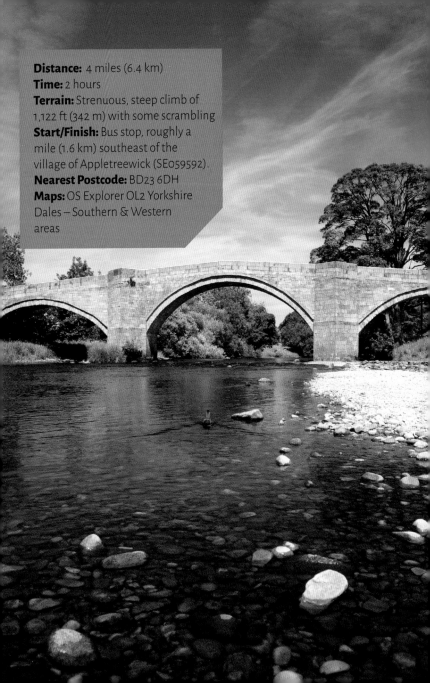

Distance: 4 miles (6.4 km)
Time: 2 hours
Terrain: Strenuous, steep climb of 1,122 ft (342 m) with some scrambling
Start/Finish: Bus stop, roughly a mile (1.6 km) southeast of the village of Appletreewick (SE059592).
Nearest Postcode: BD23 6DH
Maps: OS Explorer OL2 Yorkshire Dales – Southern & Western areas

Parking near the start of the walk is very limited, so if you can get there by bus or bike that is best. Alternatively you can park in Appletreewick and walk the mile or so to the start via Main Street and then Stangs Lane. The walk proper starts at Haugh Mill bus stop.

1 From the bus stop on Stangs Lane, head west along the sandy lane into Howgill.

2 Go left along the farm lane, passing the camp site, and continue along the lane for 1¼ miles (2 km). This is Howgill Lane, an old through route to Pateley Bridge.

3 About 100 metres short of Dalehead Farm, go through a gate on the right and climb the path which winds its way up the bracken-covered hillside for another 160 metres.

4 Cross a level track and, still climbing, bear right past an oak tree. Look for the occasional yellow arrow painted onto the rocks.

5 Scramble leftwards for about 100 metres to the trig point on the rocky summit of Simon's Seat, and take time to enjoy the magnificent views, particularly to the northwest over the village of Appletreewick and up Wharfedale.

6 Turn right, away from the rocks, and follow the steadily descending path across the moor as indicated by a signpost to Howgill and Barden, for a distance of 1 mile (1.6 km).

7 Bear right, downhill, on a rocky path and through a plantation of pine trees.

8 Cross Howgill Lane and rejoin the track down to the road bridge.

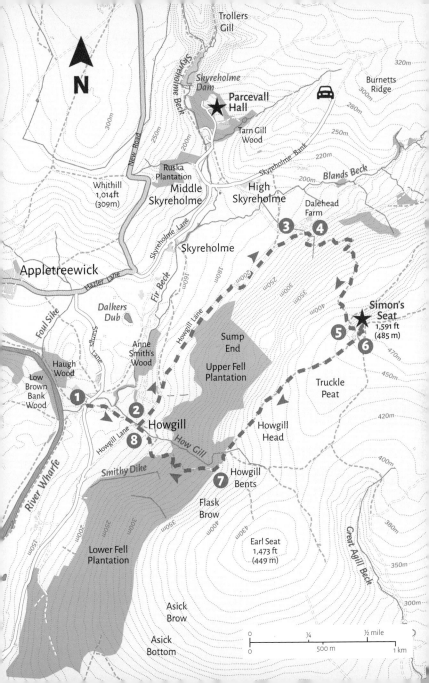

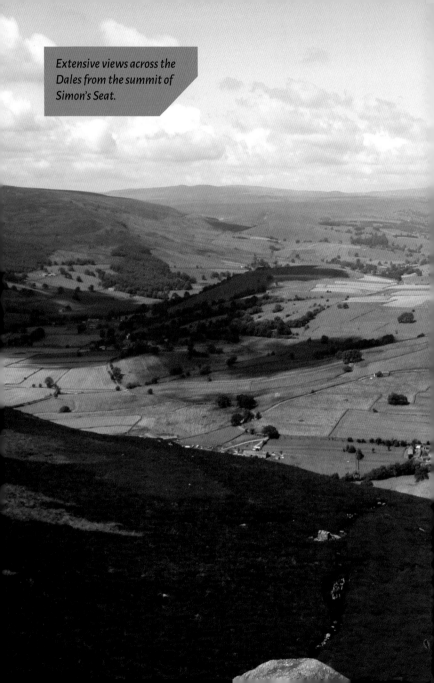

Extensive views across the Dales from the summit of Simon's Seat.

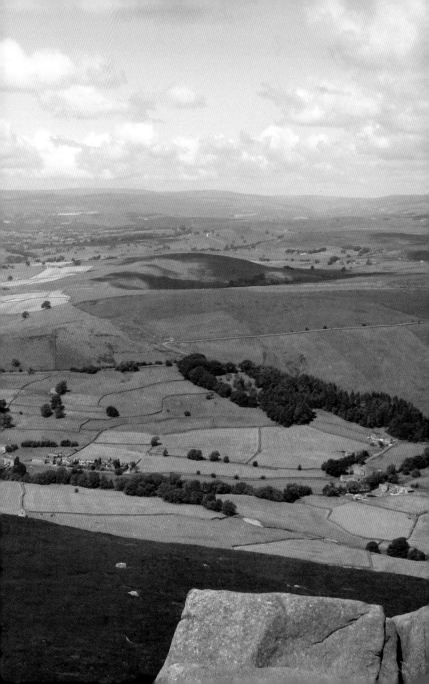

WALK 18

Attermire Scar

Explore this limestone wonderland, which was once roamed by mammoths and rhinoceros.

The busy market town of Settle, the 'capital' of Upper Ribblesdale, is the starting point for this circular walk, which takes you to a fascinating area of rocky outcrops high above the town. Once at the top, the path follows the base of a limestone scar system that extends for over a mile (1.6 km) in length. As well as being an impressive landform in itself, the scar contains a series of caves, the largest of which is Victoria Cave, named in 1837 in honour of the new Queen.

The limestone of this area was laid down in shallow seas close to the equator about 340 million years ago. It is difficult to imagine a more different environment to where the rock is found now, but archeological excavations in Victoria Cave have revealed animal bone remains that help to illustrate the more recent sequence of environmental changes, from the hippos and spotted hyenas of warm periods to the brown bears and reindeer of the last ice age. Evidence of human activity has also been found in the cave, including a 11,000-year-old barbed harpoon point made from deer antler, and Roman coins and brooches.

Due to the dangerously unstable roof, it is not recommended for people to explore inside Victoria Cave.

There are a range of facilities in Settle and several car parks. The town can be reached by train and is well served by buses.

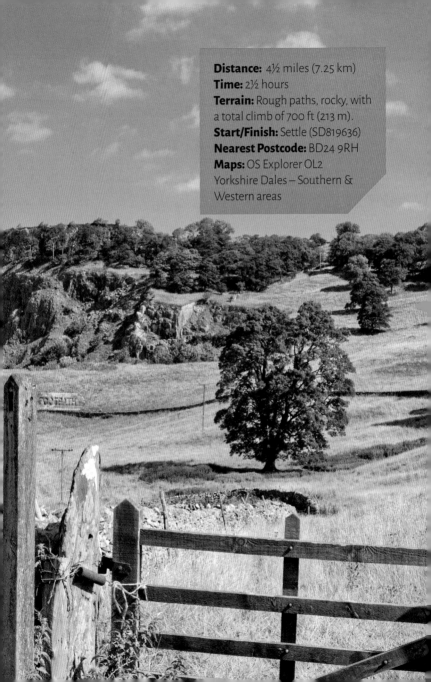

Distance: 4½ miles (7.25 km)
Time: 2½ hours
Terrain: Rough paths, rocky, with a total climb of 700 ft (213 m).
Start/Finish: Settle (SD819636)
Nearest Postcode: BD24 9RH
Maps: OS Explorer OL2 Yorkshire Dales – Southern & Western areas

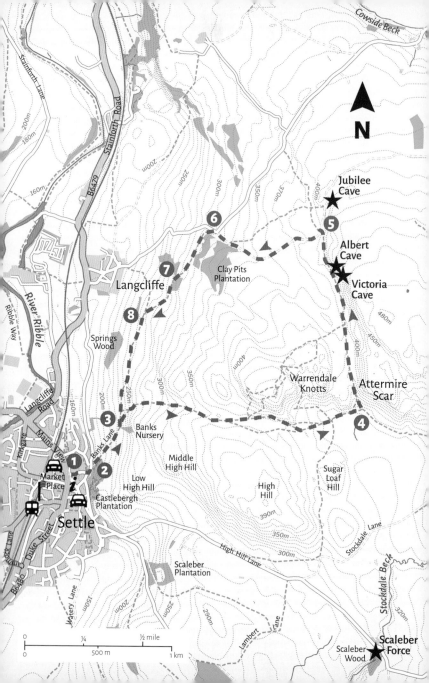

1 From the market place in the centre of Settle, walk up the road named Constitution Hill for about 150 metres.

2 Bear right, away from the road and follow the rough-walled lane uphill.

3 About 100 metres beyond a clump of trees, turn right at a signpost to Malham and climb the grassy hillside. At first, there is no path but one soon develops. Follow this to the right of the boundary wall until you reach the base of Attermire Scar.

4 Cross a stile and then go through a gap in the wall. Turn left and climb the rocky path along the foot of the scar for a little over ¾ mile (1.2 km).

5 Turn left through a metal gate and follow the well-made farm track downhill.

6 At the point where the track joins the road, turn left through a small gate and follow a field path along the bottom edge of a mature wood.

7 Pass through the gate in the narrow gap between two sections of woodland.

8 Take the stile at the side of the wicket gate. Walk ahead along a field path and descend by an improving track, retracing your steps back into Settle for the final part of the walk.

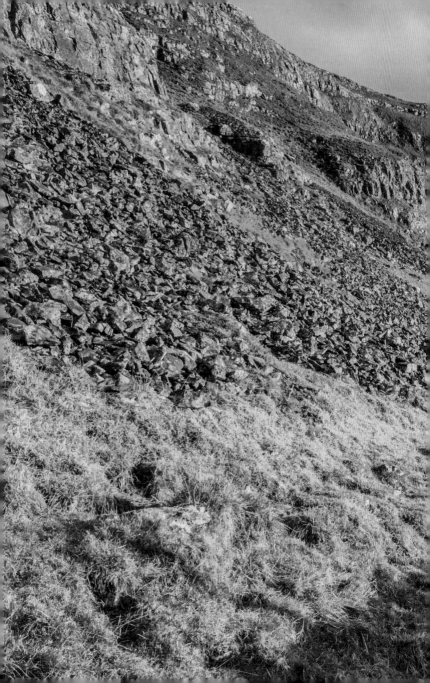

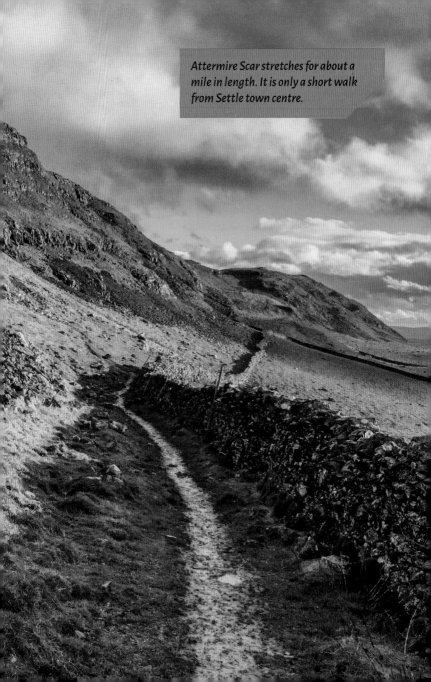

Attermire Scar stretches for about a mile in length. It is only a short walk from Settle town centre.

WALK 19
Pen-y-ghent

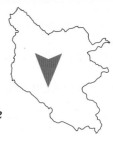

Climb up through the geological time scale on this classic Dales mountain.

Most of the Pennine summits are high points in areas of upland moorland, but the graceful mountain of Pen-y-ghent is a real peak. It rises above the town of Horton in Ribblesdale, which is the usual starting point for the gruelling race, or individual attempts, on the Yorkshire Three Peaks. This challenge involves covering a distance of 24 miles (38.6 km) and a total ascent of 5,200 ft (1,585 m) while taking on the peaks of Pen-y-ghent, Whernside and Ingleborough.

This circular walk takes you to the summit of the smallest of the Three Peaks, whose name could mean 'hill on the border'. It is an ideal place to introduce children to mountain climbing; they might agree that when viewed from a distance, the domed outline of Pen-y-ghent forms the shape of a crouching lion.

The mountain has clear horizontal rock strata, with carboniferous limestones at the base, which are overlaid with sandstones and shales and capped with millstone grit. The rocks on the steep southern side were exposed in great rakes when a tremendous thunderstorm washed away the topsoil in 1881.

Approaching the peak from the south, the route follows part of the Pennine Way over the summit and down the steep slope past Hunt Pot cave entrance, before heading back into Horton in Ribblesdale. All facilities are available in the village, which is served by both buses and trains.

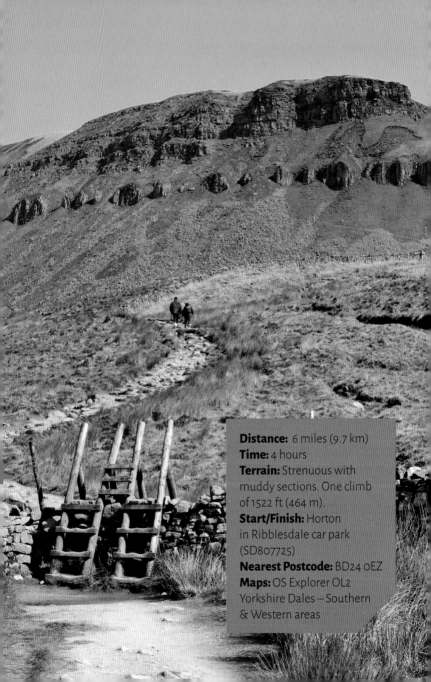

Distance: 6 miles (9.7 km)
Time: 4 hours
Terrain: Strenuous with muddy sections. One climb of 1522 ft (464 m).
Start/Finish: Horton in Ribblesdale car park (SD807725)
Nearest Postcode: BD24 0EZ
Maps: OS Explorer OL2 Yorkshire Dales – Southern & Western areas

1 The walk starts at the car park on the B6479 diagonally opposite the Crown Hotel in Horton in Ribblesdale. Walk south, past the church and then left on a side road following Douk Ghyll stream.

2 Turn left at Brackenbottom Farm and follow the signposted footpath uphill for a distance of 1 mile (1.6 km), crossing all walls by their stiles.

3 Climb over the stile and turn left to join the Pennine Way path, which you follow steeply uphill. Scramble though the craggy gritstone outcrops and follow the wide path towards the summit cairn.

4 Climb the ladder stile to reach the summit, taking time to enjoy the stunning views. Leave by a wide path, which slants to the right, and takes you down the rocky slope for ½ mile (800 m).

5 Turn sharp left at the path junction and go steeply down towards the boggy moor, passing the surface fissure of Hunt Pot.

6 Turn left through a gate at the side of a ruined shooting cabin. Follow the walled lane downhill for 1½ miles (2.4 km).

7 The lane joins the B6479 conveniently close to the Pen-y-ghent Café. Turn right along the road to return to the car park on the left.

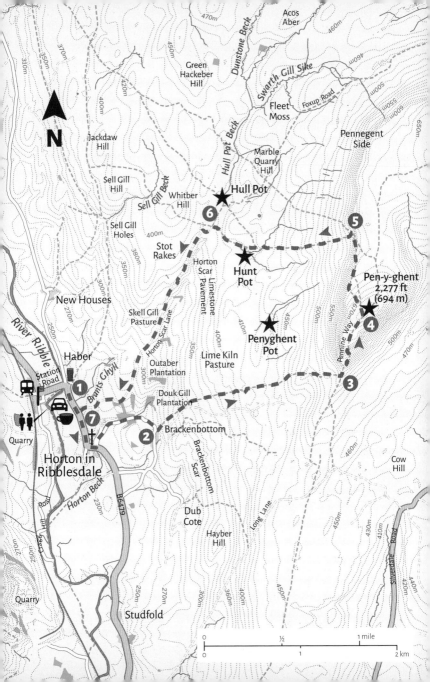

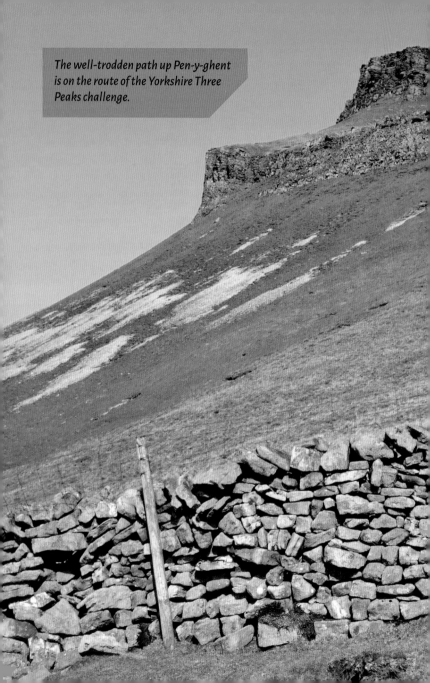

The well-trodden path up Pen-y-ghent is on the route of the Yorkshire Three Peaks challenge.

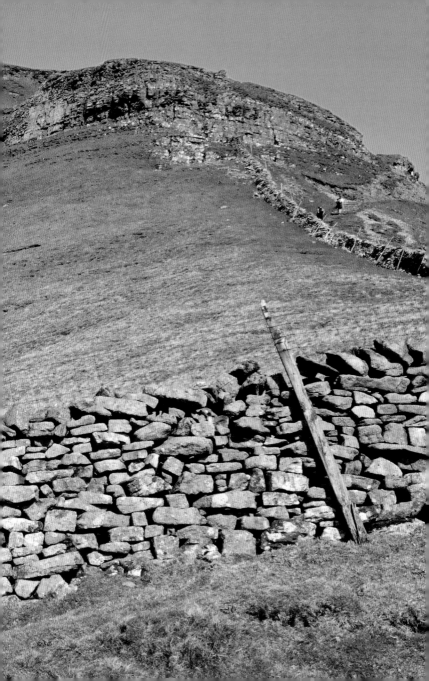

WALK 20
Chapel-le-Dale

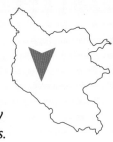

An easy walk for all weathers, in the valley between the Dales' two highest mountains.

Nestled in the valley between the towering masses of Ingleborough and Whernside, the tiny village of Chapel-le-Dale sits on the route of the Cam High Road, the Roman road linking nearby Ingleton with the fort at Bainbridge.

The 'chapel in the valley' after which the village is named is St Leonard's Church, a chapel of ease serving the residents who were unable to journey to their parish church at Low Bentham, 8 miles (13 km) away, for regular worship. The charming chapel was constructed in the seventeenth century, of limestone, and incorporates several beautiful stained-glass windows. If the churchyard seems large for such a small community, it is because it served as the final resting place for over 200 railway workers and their families who died during construction of the Settle to Carlisle railway. There are memorials to them both inside and outside the church.

This circular walk from the village makes use of farm lanes and roads for its entire length, making it a suitable route for all weather conditions. The scenery in the dale is stunning, with both mountainsides tiered with limestone scars, and potholes in the valley bottom, the most well-known of which – Hurtle Pot – is, according to folklore, home to an evil spirit called a boggart.

You will pass a pub as you return to the village, otherwise facilities are available in Ingleton, 4 miles (7 km) away.

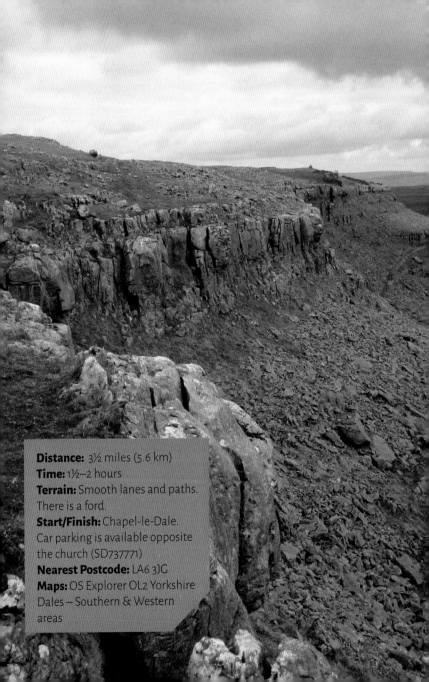

Distance: 3½ miles (5.6 km)
Time: 1½–2 hours
Terrain: Smooth lanes and paths.
There is a ford.
Start/Finish: Chapel-le-Dale.
Car parking is available opposite
the church (SD737771)
Nearest Postcode: LA6 3JG
Maps: OS Explorer OL2 Yorkshire
Dales – Southern & Western
areas

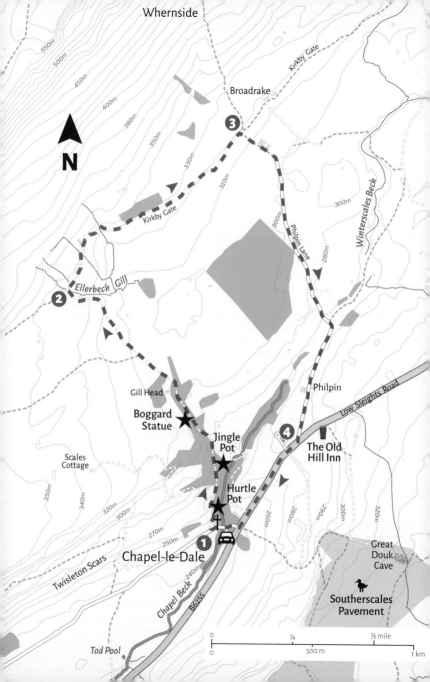

1 Park near St Leonard's Church in Chapel-le-Dale. Turn right behind the church and follow the wooded lane uphill for a mile (1.6 km), passing Hurtle Pot and Jingle Pot, which are potholes linked to the same flooded cave system. Look out for the boggart statue on the left.

2 Cross the shallow ford at Ellerbeck and follow the farm lane to the right. Go through the farmyard and out along a cart track to the right for a little under a mile (1.6 km).

3 Turn right at a signpost marked 'Hill Inn'. Go down the surfaced lane.

4 At the main road, refreshment is available about (165 m) to the left at The Old Hill Inn. Otherwise, follow the road to the right as far as the side road on your right, turning into Chapel-le-Dale.

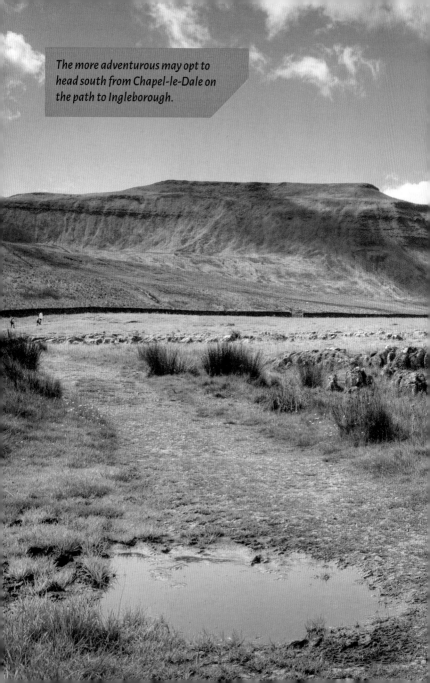

The more adventurous may opt to head south from Chapel-le-Dale on the path to Ingleborough.

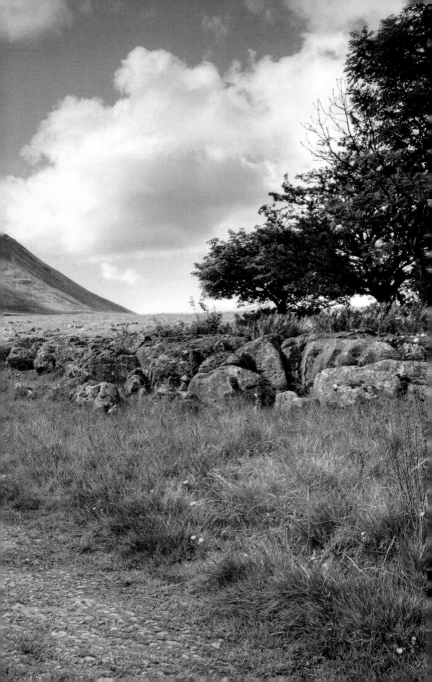

Acknowledgements

Thanks to all of the photographers who allowed us to use their imagery in this book.

page 6 © Stephen Garnett; 9 © Dan Kay; 12 © Wendy McDonnell; 19 © Mark Sadler; 22-23 © Mark Sadler; 25 © Dan Cook; 29 © Christopher Werrett; 33 © Mark Sadler; 36-37 © Mark Sadler; 39 © Andy Kay; 42 © Andy Kay; 45 © Christopher Werrett; 48-49 © Christopher Werrett; 51 © Paul Harris; 54-55 © Paul Harris; 57 © Andy Kay; 61 © Paul Harris; 64-65 © Paul Harris; 67 © Christopher Werrett; 71 © Matt Sullivan; 74-75 © Jeremy George; 77 © andrew j w; 80-81 © Jez Campbell/Shutterstock;83 © Tom Curtis/Shutterstock; 86-87 © Tom Curtis/Shutterstock; 89 © Gutsibikes; 92-93 © Kevin Eaves/Shutterstock; 95 © Matt Sullivan; 98-99 © westy48; 101 © Matt Sullivan; 105 © pwhittle/Shutterstock; 108-109 © George Green/Shutterstock; 111 © Kevin Eaves/Shutterstock; 114-115 © Pete Stuart/Shutterstock; 117 © Kevin Eaves/Shutterstock; 120-121 © Kevin Eaves/Shutterstock; 123 © Nicholas Peter Gavin Davies/ Shutterstock; 126-127 © Kevin Eaves/Shutterstock

Maps © OpenStreetMap contributors
Contains OS data © Crown copyright [and database right] 2020.
Map creation: Cosmographics Ltd (www.cosmographics.co.uk).
Page design and layout: mapuccino (mapuccino.com.au).
Edited by Karen Marland.